CL16

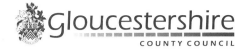
Gloucestershire
COUNTY COUNCIL

Items should be returned to any Gloucestershire County Library
on or before the date stamped. Books which are not in demand may
be renewed in person, by letter or telephone.
0845 230 5420

D0279447

The SuperStress Solution

Roberta Lee, M.D.

BANTAM PRESS

LONDON • TORONTO • SYDNEY • AUCKLAND • JOHANNESBURG

TRANSWORLD PUBLISHERS
61–63 Uxbridge Road, London W5 5SA
A Random House Group Company
www.rbooks.co.uk

First published in the United States
in 2010 by Random House,
an imprint of The Random House Publishing Group,
a division of Random House, Inc., New York

First published in Great Britain
in 2010 by Bantam Press
an imprint of Transworld Publishers

Design by BTD NYC

A CIP catalogue record for this book
is available from the British Library.

ISBN 9780593061886

The author has changed the names and identifying characteristics of some of the
individuals whose medical cases are discussed in this book. Any resemblance to real
persons, living or dead, is entirely coincidental and unintentional.

No book can replace the diagnostic expertise and medical advice of a trusted
doctor. Please be certain to consult with your doctor before making any decisions
that affect your health, particularly if you suffer from any medical condition or
have any symptom that may require treatment.

Addresses for Random House Group Ltd companies outside the UK
can be found at: www.randomhouse.co.uk
The Random House Group Ltd Reg. No. 954009

The Random House Group Limited supports the Forest Stewardship
Council (FSC), the leading international forest-certification organization. All our
titles that are printed on Greenpeace-approved FSC-certified paper carry the FSC logo.
Our paper procurement policy can be found at www.rbooks.co.uk/environment

Printed and bound in Great Britain by
Clays Ltd, Bungay Suffolk

2 4 6 8 10 9 7 5 3 1

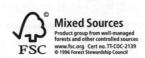

Mixed Sources
Product group from well-managed
forests and other controlled sources
www.fsc.org   Cert no. TT-COC-2139
© 1996 Forest Stewardship Council
FSC

Contents

Introduction

A NEW KIND OF STRESS, A NEW SOLUTION

I'M TAPPING THIS OUT on my laptop under the sole lightbulb in the dark jet bringing me home to New York from my monthlong stay on the islands of Micronesia. I first went to these coral reef islands in 1988 when, as a newly minted physician fresh out of residency, I joined the U.S. Public Health Service and was immediately dispatched there for five years. My task then was to provide Western medical care to those who needed it and, when necessary, to bring the islanders to the main island for more intensive treatment. For the past nine years, I've returned there for a month every year to do research with traditional healers, studying their vision of health and illness, as well as learning about their use of herbal medicines. Much of what I learned and observed there has informed my medical practice today. I continue to be awed by the methods and philosophies of these indigenous healers.

Tonight, as the drone of the engines pulses steadily through the cabin, I feel that all of my fellow passengers are asleep. I wish that hum could lull me into oblivion so I could tune out at least some of the twenty grueling hours that remain of the flight. But I can't sleep—and not just because I'm cramped in my airline seat. I can't because a nagging ache that started at the base of my neck is now radiating down to the muscles between my shoulder blades. It used to appear a month or so after I returned home, but now it shows up sharply and acutely just a couple of hours into my return flight. I think I know why.

With each passing year, my New York life grows exponentially more hectic and demanding, and I know what's facing me almost as soon as I get off the plane. As a doctor, I must respond and react far more swiftly now than I did a decade ago—and at all hours of the day and night. My patients expect this, as they, too, seem to be caught up in their own frenetic worlds. Also, I know all too well that the serenity that I have just enjoyed throughout my monthlong stay on the islands—a serenity I have grown to cherish—will be gone the moment I unbuckle my seat belt.

In Micronesia, no matter how hard I work—and some days I go nonstop from dawn to dusk—at the end of the day I always feel a sense of peace and tranquility. And yet each time I return to the States, I see the tranquility gap between here and there widen. While the islanders seem suspended in a state of calm, I and my patients back home in New York City, where I have lived for many years, are getting more and more frenzied.

And here is something else: Not only do my patients appear more stressed; they have started describing symptoms of stress at *increasingly younger ages*. It used to be that most people in the waiting rooms of general practitioners were there for treatment of diseases associated with aging, such as diabetes, high blood pressure, and heart disease. They were in their fifties, sixties, and older. And yet my patient population has been heading in the other direction. It now includes a growing number of thirty- and forty-year-olds.

I also see a whole new battery of complaints creeping into patient histories, from young to old. Some people come to me knowing that they are terribly stressed, but not really sure why or what to do about it. Others come in describing what we now know are stress-induced illnesses. And yet, when I ask them whether they are feeling stressed, they tell me they're not. "I'm not sure what it is, Doctor," said one patient who practically dragged himself into my office. "But I know I've got *something* because I'm not sleeping. I'm exhausted. Energy's gone . . . along with my sex drive." Another patient, a woman in her late thirties, a commodities trader whose office was very near where the World Trade Center had been, came in with a terrible case of hives on her chest and forehead caused, she told me, by nothing she could put her finger on. She only knew that she was anxious all the time. When I asked about what might be stressing her—other than her high-stress job—she stoically told me that nothing was any different from the usual. It hadn't even occurred to her that her proximity to a place that had known such catastrophe might be psychologically weighing on her.

These two people are hardly isolated cases. I regularly see any number of patients who are plagued with irritable anxiety, substance abuse, sleep disorders, and withdrawal from life. Many come in bewildered by what they are experiencing—everything from strange digestive, allergic, respiratory, sexual, and skin problems to autoimmune dysfunction and heart disease. And yes. Some patients do understand what's happening enough to complain, "I'm so stressed out!" But the great majority has no idea that stress is playing a significant or catalyzing role in their afflictions. All they know is that they've slipped over an edge; that they've caught something that won't go away.

A NEW KIND OF STRESS, A NEW SOLUTION

What they've "caught" is a menacing form of stress that closely resembles post-traumatic stress disorder (PTSD). Known as "shell shock" when it was first identified after World War I, PTSD usually stems from a catastrophic life event—combat, rape, involvement with a deadly accident, or a major illness—that leaves its victim in a persistent highly anxious state that leads to disengagement from life, sleep disorders, and substance abuse habits that are so elevated as to place them in a new category on the diagnostic scale. After the original distress and emotional fallout, many victims gradually return to life as usual. But not all. For some, the stress—and the memories—persist. Occasionally, PTSD sufferers re-experience the traumatic event or events through flashbacks or nightmares and, as a result, they tend to avoid places, people, or other things that remind them of the event. They remain off-balance, their bodies literally in an I'm-at-war mode all the time. But most of my patients haven't suffered through the experiences that are so often linked to PTSD, yet their symptoms are very much the same.

What's going on?

About a decade ago, I decided to keep a closer eye on a group of patients who had been exhibiting a number of physical symptoms that more often than not came in multiples. They denied experiencing any unusual stress in their lives. After I talked with them for hours on end, it came to me one day, right out of the blue: *These people had been living with extreme stress for so long that they didn't even realize they were stressed!* They had crossed the line from a pale shade of gray to a very deep dark black state in their bodies, but they hadn't noticed the transformation. Stress had become an invisible part of the landscape of their lives.

And it wasn't just job stress. They had job stress *and* money stress *and* parenting stress *and* relationship stress *and* trying-to-find-a-taxi-in-the-rain stress. Layers upon layers of stress weighed on them in increments so small that they didn't feel them separately. Here, right under my nose, was an insidious new threat to everyone's well-being, a menacing, twenty-first-century kind of stress that, because it was above and beyond anything I had ever seen before, I gave the name *SuperStress*.

It's not your grandmother's stress, that's for sure.

I don't mean to imply that any specific event—not even 9/11—caused this epidemic. Not at all. What I think is that the pace of life has escalated so radically during this decade that we can no longer fool ourselves into thinking that we're living the lives of our grandparents—or even of our parents. The twenty-first century is barely a decade old, yet it is already posing new and dangerous challenges that many of us not only welcome but also actually seek out.

Just consider the advances in the technology we use every day. Between cell phones, handheld computers, and new communication modes like texting and Twittering, we're "on call" and open to intrusion twenty-four hours a day. One recent survey commissioned by support.com reported that 40 percent of eighteen-to-twenty-five-year-old students said they couldn't cope without their cell phones. And yet, when they stopped using them for three days—as the study asked them to do—these students reported less stress and had lower heart rates and blood pressure.[1] And, then, of course, there's the computer. Most of us spend long hours every day staring at flickering monitors, ever alert to emails and instant messages that demand quick replies. That same survey of over a thousand people found that 65 percent of respondents spent more time with their computer than with their spouse or significant other. More than 80 percent of those polled said they were more dependent on their computer today than they were three years ago.

Technology isn't the only offender, either. Noise pollution, even in the smallest towns, can cause stress in a major way. Have you ever pulled up to a red light and found yourself alongside a car that's blasting its music so loud that *your* car begins to vibrate? Your choices are to a) run the red light, or b) sit there and take it. Have you ever sat down in a coffee shop for an eagerly anticipated catch-up lunch with a friend, only to find that the young woman sitting at the very next table is having a catch-up lunch with *her* friend? Only there's no one else at her table; she's loudly crossing the miles on her cell phone. For Shakespeare, all the world was a stage. Today, all the world is a telephone booth.

Television has been our electronic hearth for decades, but it, too, has changed. Today's not-so-small-screen programming unfolds at speeds that make our heads spin. We're blitzed with fast-paced sensory stimulation whenever we turn it on, and our nervous systems respond with a rush of arousal. Stepped-up-volume commercials change images as fast as MTV videos do, and we never give it a second thought. We just sit and listen, numbed to the outside world. Today, TV sets are everywhere. A decade ago there was never a television screen in your bank. But now there is. You can watch *Oprah* in your local coffee shop, CNN at the airport, and the sitcom du jour in the back of your New York City taxicab. There's probably a TV in your dentist's waiting room and one in his examining room. You can get your teeth cleaned while you watch Judge Judy mediate between dueling spouses. (Talk about multitasking!)

Professional and personal expectations have risen exponentially as well. In a culture that downplays long-term thinking in favor of constant, measurable productivity, our employers set frequent, must-hit benchmarks that we must, of course, hit—or else. With tough competition for slots at top schools, parents feel overwhelming pressure to manage their kids' every move, often at the expense of their own downtime as well as their child's. Does five-year-old Sammy really need to be in chess club? He does if he buys into his parents' fear that he might not be smart enough in thirteen years to get into an Ivy. (Welcome to the next generation of SuperStressed individuals.)

Add to these daily challenges and intrusions the cultural backdrop: a 24/7 news cycle that keeps us edgy with Code Orange and Code Red terror alerts; cynical corruption in Washington; devastating wars in Afghanistan and Iraq; threats of bird and swine flu, anthrax, ricin, and lethal strains of staph; gunmen on the rampage in schools, workplaces, and shopping malls; mass-transit bombings in Madrid and London; the tragedy of Darfur; martial law in nuclear-armed Pakistan—and the list goes on and on.

Biologically, the human species hasn't evolved beyond "island time," that is, the slower pace of life on the island. And yet we're expected to increase the pace of our activity by orders of magnitude just to keep up. We can't do it. Not without paying a price. And that's because the hardwiring of our brains and bodies is the same as it was in the days of our ancestors, even while change accelerates all around us. For example:

Our food sources have changed. It's no secret that our food is moving farther and farther away from its natural form. Pick up a small packet of beef bouillon the next time you're in a supermarket and try reading the list of ingredients out loud. It's a good thing that the FDA has determined by law that foods post their ingredients on the package, but there are few limitations to that list of ingredients. And our food choices have changed along with the availability of fast—and even of gourmet—foods. (Don't get me started on portion sizes.)

Our daily sleep-wake rhythms have shifted. Few of us wake up when the sun rises and go to sleep when the sun sets. We're rising before the sun to get to the gym because there's no time to work out later in the day. And we're up working at all hours of the night because our jobs rarely finish at a normal hour. Even if we do go to sleep well before midnight, in many cases ambient streetlight makes its way into our bedrooms and disturbs our natural circadian rhythm.

Our job satisfaction seems to be rapidly eroding. There are many reasons for this, one being the number of roles our society allows most men and women to choose from. While we enjoy the variety and the opportunity to choose, we also face the complexity that comes with them. Perhaps we're attempting to fill too many roles when our basic human nature is to have one: to either provide or protect, to either nurture or feed.

In our urban workplaces, the fear of being laid off has reached epidemic proportions. *Downsizing*—a word that decades ago was known only to business school graduates and CEOs—has become all too familiar. So has *outsourcing*. And the human factor in many of the jobs that we do have doesn't seem to be the kind of human relationship that really gives us pleasure back. In other words, small pleasant conversations at the grocery store or coffee shop are all too rare these days. I recently went to a fast-food chain and ordered a sandwich and coffee. The server behind the counter took my order, typing it into the computer as I spoke. She put together my sandwich, dispensed the coffee from an enormous vat, placed both in a paper bag, secured the top, handed the bag to me, took my money, gave me change, and all the while *never looked up*. In Micronesia, where it's rude to have any kind of transaction in which there isn't at least eye contact, this behavior would be unthinkable.

WE'RE DELUDING OURSELVES if we think that we can indefinitely endure the macro stresses that accompany impersonal encounters, less sleep, more work, less leisure, raising kids in this dangerous world, bad marriages, less exercise, junk and processed foods eaten on the run, hyper-caffeinated and sugar-saturated beverages, addictive devices that give us "screen sickness," traffic jams, flight delays, and so much more, and come away unscathed. Each one of these situations carries with it a hit to our nervous system, and a collection of such hits literally jackhammers us right into SuperStress. The bottom line: our nervous system is not designed to take that kind of beating.

We as a species have evolved to handle short-term stress situations. We can even endure, if we must, some fairly longer-term stress, such as a bad marriage or a stack of overdue bills when there's nothing left in the bank account. But all stress all the time changes the nature of this into a different disease. This is the one I call SuperStress.

SuperStress is not just a matter of so many jangled nerves. It's a new pandemic, as deadly as any public health crisis we have ever faced.

In the last half of the twentieth century a large majority of health issues were related to cigarette smoking, and there was an all-out blitz to get people to give up the habit. That was followed by a decade or so of what came to be known as a fat epidemic. With a high incidence of obesity endemic to our society, medical science has been trying every which way to stem the tide before diseases like diabetes affect as much as 50 percent of our population.

But this is century twenty-one, folks. Today, much of the scientific interest has shifted from fat to stress—and not a moment too soon. You'll see as we get further into the book that stress is at the base of as many if not more diseases than are associated with obesity. But while obesity is easily diagnosed—let's face it, you know it when you see it—stress has no face. It hides insidiously behind illnesses of its own making. Any doctor—indigenous, conventional, integrative, or functional—will tell you the same thing if you are continually stressed and you don't deal with it: *this kind of stress can kill you.*

BUT HERE'S THE GOOD NEWS: it doesn't have to.

THE SUPERSTRESS SOLUTION

Take heart. I'm not going to suggest that you move to an island in the South Pacific. Nor am I going to suggest that you remove yourself from every stressful situation you encounter, because we both know that in this day and age, it's clearly impossible. (Let's be honest, here. Are you going to quit your stressful job? No. Are your children never going to worry or challenge you? You wish.)

Rather, the resolution lies in a new paradigm for health—an easy-to-use approach to your well-being that I call the *SuperStress Solution.* Some of the traditional therapies that I learned and embraced in Micronesia find a place in the solution, as do the integrative modalities that I learned as one of four physicians in the first graduating class at Dr. Andrew Weil's famed Program in Integrative Medicine in Arizona. Put those together with things I have learned since then in my own integrative practice in New York, and you've got my holistic prescription. It's all here, in this book that you are holding in your hands right now.

After more comprehensively defining SuperStress in a scientific sense in Chapter 1, I invite you to take the robust questionnaires on pages 42–50. This will help you pinpoint your own level of SuperStress and begin to see patterns of when it strikes you most often and how it manifests in your daily behavior. What are you giving up when you remain in a SuperStressed state? You'll find that out, too.

Part 2 of my plan defines what I call the tools for change, a series of six different SuperStress-busting, lifestyle-enhancing tools that are the foundation of the Four-Week SuperStress Solution, week-by-week details of which you'll find laid out for you in Part 3. If, however, you are like many of my patients and would prefer to spot treat your stress-related symptoms, I also offer you specific quick-fix solutions in the "SuperStress Solutions for Your Type" chapter starting on page 209. Attending to the most obvious or serious of your stress-related symptoms in this way may be just what you need to ratchet down your stress enough to begin taking a longer view. At that point, I hope you'll consider the four-week program as well.

If you are looking for proven life-changing benefits—from clearer thinking to better relationships in love, family, friendship and work, increased efficiency, more joy and laughter, and better general health—the Four-Week SuperStress Solution will help you do just that. It offers twenty-first-century treatments for a twenty-first-century ailment and will, in effect, retrain your nervous system to default to a state of rest. It will teach you to shut down the stress circuit and relax deeply.

My program, rooted in the principles of integrative medicine, is designed to teach you how to control your thoughts and the negative emotions that are so closely associated with SuperStress. You'll be able to identify exactly how you feel when you feel your best and most relaxed, and how you feel when you're at your worst and most stressed. You'll learn to recognize the specific circumstances that are making you feel that way, as well as how to use your mind and body to get to the good place and maintain that feeling—no matter what real and pressing problems you experience. In essence, this program is a way for you to take back control, to build access to your own private sanctuary of peace and tranquility.

Life is so much more than a series of emergencies, deadlines, mistakes, calamities waiting to happen, impossible decisions, traps, guilt, worries, and losses. And it's yours to live any way you want. Sure, I understand that letting go of your stress might seem as scary as jumping from a speeding train, but by the end of this book you'll understand why you feel stressed, and why it has become impossible for you to live even a single day with a calm mind. You've worn your stress as a badge of honor for a long time, but now it's time to give it up.

This treatment plan is divided into four one-week periods that will make the transitions to new behaviors much easier. If you want to take longer than four weeks to get through it, that's fine, too. Go at your own pace. I want you to feel empowered, not overwhelmed. None of these changes is that hard; anyone can make them. Anyone, that is, who has the insight and capacity to learn—*and the courage to change.*

So why not go for it? Why not get rid of your unnecessary stress overload—the SuperStress that's making you sick—and retrieve all the good that you know is missing from your life?

The door to your sanctuary is open. All you have to do is walk through it.

—ROBERTA LEE, M.D.

PART 1

SuperStress and You

CHAPTER ONE

SuperStress in Your Body and on Your Mind

STRESS IS A WORD WE TOSS AROUND EVERY DAY, but what does it really mean? There are probably as many definitions as there are people you ask for them. Stress is both a physiological and a psychological response to events that upset our balance. Stress is what happens when the demands and daily challenges of the outside world are greater than our ability to cope with them. But stress is related to internal factors as well—factors that include how healthy we are, our emotional well-being, what we eat, and how much sleep we get. It's also strongly dependent on how we interpret what comes our way—that is, how we perceive what's happening to us.

Each person interprets a prospectively dangerous situation differently. Let's say, for example, that six-foot-two-inch Anthony runs out of gas in the middle of a dark street in a not-so-safe neighborhood. While walking to the nearest filling station, he notices a group of four burly guys heading in his direction. He barely pays attention to them and continues on his way, never changing his pace. If his sister has the same experience with her car, when she sees the men coming her way she might a) cross the street, b) duck into the nearest open store, or c) pull out the pepper spray that she has in her handbag "just in case." For Anthony, this nonevent creates nothing more than a blip on the stress radar screen. But his sister, who perceives that she might be in danger, has a much more pronounced stress response. The stress response is about protecting ourselves and it's about having control over a situation. How much stress we feel as a result of our perception of things determines how much control we think we have.

Anything that triggers stress is known as a *stressor*. Anything that forces us to adjust to the degree that it strains our coping skills is a stressor. Stressors can range from small aggravations to fear of something or someone that might pose a threat to your well-being. Large stressors include major life events, such as a divorce, a child leaving home, an unexpected pregnancy, a move to a new town, a career change, graduating from college, or a diagnosis of cancer. But while major life changes are stressful, it's the stressors that come at us—and consequently at our nervous systems—all day long that affect us the most. These include:

- *Environmental stressors,* such as noise pollution (from blaring radios, barking dogs, or police sirens) or living in a crime-ridden neighborhood where you never feel safe.
- *Work stressors,* such as job dissatisfaction, overwork, disagreements with your boss, low pay, or nasty office politics.
- *Relationship stressors*—defined as a fight with a friend; problems with partners, children, or other family members; or loss of a spouse.
- *Social stressors* that occur when you're trying to keep up with the Joneses or trying to *be* the Joneses.
- *Spiritual angst,* which can come from loss of a purpose in your life. Loss of community. Loss of control. Loss of meaning.

FEAR AS A STRESSOR

Fear is one of the great stressors of all time. Fear heralds many dangers and yet it can save us by keeping us in fight-or-flight mode. Our ancestors—long ago—had no choice but to be faster, stronger, and more cunning than the predators that waited for them to make a mistake. The fact is, a guy going out alone on the savanna in search of food knew well that when he came face-to-face with a beast, he was either going to get lunch or *be* lunch. In those days, if you didn't have enough you were going to die of starvation or hypothermia. If you were successful, you might be alone. The last one standing. And *then* what?

Today, our fears are more socially related and can almost always be broken into different categories: fear of failure, fear of not having enough, fear of not being enough, fear of losing what you've got, fear of success. Do I have enough to keep up with the neighbors? Am I pretty enough for the guy I have a crush on? It seems almost banal to label some of these trivial things "fears," but the threats are very real to the person who experiences them. The problem is that the brain doesn't understand enough to think: *Are you kidding me? You call this a threat or a danger?* The brain interprets fear as *Oh, my God, we're under siege!* It immediately signals a meant-to-be-protective cascade of hormones: epinephrine, or epinephrine and cortisol. So whether you fall off a cliff or dream you're falling off a cliff, your neurological response will be precisely the same.

Stressors are cumulative, so the more life changes or daily hassles you're dealing with at any one time, the more intense the symptoms of stress. With our twenty-first-century lifestyle, the hassle factor of everyday life has grown exponentially. Bear in mind that a series of small hassles can eventually combine to become several dangerous ones.

CHRONIC STRESS AND THE LOAD YOU CARRY

Our bodies are hardwired to respond to stress the same way our ancestors did, and under acute conditions that response did (and still does) protect us. It helped our ancestors out of dangerous situations when the best course of action was to literally get out of harm's way. Acute stress can have positive benefits. It has been shown to improve certain body systems, such as the immune system. The skin is more able to fight infection and our five senses and short-term memory are often enhanced during acute stress situations. However, in today's world, most of the stress we feel is in response to chronic rather than acute threats. Unfortunately, the brain, for all its majesty, can't distinguish acute from chronic. In that respect, it's a lot like Chicken Little, assuming the worst-case scenario every time it senses a threat. And when the stress doesn't go away—when your project deadline is two weeks away and that seems like less than half the time you need to complete it—then the hormones dispatched by the brain in an effort to mount a defense just keep coming. Dr. Bruce McEwen of Rockefeller University, an expert on the physiological effects of chronic stress, describes this crossover from acute to chronic stress as a journey from *allostasis* to *allostatic load.*

Allostasis is the body's way of keeping all systems in balance, particularly as we move from one situation to another. For example, climbing stairs sets our heart working harder for the extra effort our legs need, but at the top of the stairs, the pumping slows down again. The same adjustments work when you leave your walk in the snow and head inside for a chat by the fire; your body temperature automatically adjusts itself. Last example: Imagine you are crossing the street. You see an out-of-control car coming at you; your brain senses the danger and thinks, *Get out of the way!* In a split second, your body produces stress hormones that fuel your sprint to the other side of the street and safety. Ten minutes later, the incident is all but forgotten and you're happily trying on shoes in Target. Your stress hormones, no longer needed, have stopped surging and all systems are back to normal. This is allostasis in its finest hour.

It's one thing to dash across a street to avoid an oncoming car, but when there are too many such threats in a relatively short period of time or when any one stressor goes on too long—as when a person stays in a bad marriage—then we begin carrying what is known as an allostatic load. If allostasis is the body's ability to maintain balance under stress, allostatic load refers to the factors that threaten to destabilize it.

McEwen cites several different types of allostatic load:[1]

1) *When multiple stressors lead to elevated stress hormones that continue over a long period of time.* Perhaps you lost your job, and as a result had to sell your car, can't afford your mortgage payments, and to top it all off you have to explain to the kids why they can't go to camp this year.

2) *When you can't seem to adapt to a stressor even though it repeats itself again and again.* Let's say you're one of the many people terrified by the thought of public speaking. You've been invited to present at a prestigious conference and so you suck it up, feel the stress—and give a great talk. It goes so well that you're asked to make the same presentation at ten other events. If you fail to adapt

to the stress—if you're just as scared the tenth time as the first—that situation is going to register as allostatic load.

3) *When your body turns on the stress hormones and doesn't turn them off after the stressor has gone.* In other words, you experience too much stress to cope with in a given time. For example: You have a conflict at work that has been resolved, and yet when you come home that night you're still agitated, replaying the conversation over and over again in your head.

These examples all showcase forms of chronic stress, and over the years, we've all had our share. But today's society has increased chronic stressors to assault proportions, and we're left dealing with the fallout. We're surrounded by technology, all-news-all-the-time, noise pollution, job stress, unnatural food, in-office competition, relationship and parenting challenges—all coming at us from all sides, 24/7/365. It's a relentless attack that permeates to the bones. It's allostatic load—only more so. While stress in the old days was an annoyance that you eventually could manage—kind of like a gnat flying around your head—today's stress is like a bullhorn that's two inches away from your ear. Today's stress is the kind of stress that defaults your nervous system to agitation rather than rest, with serious consequences for both mind and body.

ACCUMULATED CHRONIC STRESS—SUPERSTRESS

Today's stress is of such magnitude that it can only be called *SuperStress*. The levels of complexity in SuperStress are much more insidious than we've ever seen in chronic stress. SuperStress is layers and layers of stress piled atop one another so subtly that sometimes we don't even notice what's happening.

SuperStress is damaging to the body in many ways. For one, continuous or repeated surges of stress hormones are detrimental to the cardiovascular and immune systems, potentially increasing your risk of coronary heart disease, stroke, cancer, recurrent infection, and other chronic diseases. For another, you are more likely to turn to destructive behaviors to deal with it—such as excessive smoking, drinking, or overeating. Finally, the more often the stress response is activated, the harder it becomes to shut off, so that eventually you find yourself responding to a relatively mild stressor as if it were a life-threatening one. Less is more, but not in a good way.

This latter point was brought home recently when I had dinner with an old college friend I hadn't seen in years. We were on our second course when she started to tell me about her niece, Laura, a young woman of twenty-nine who had just returned from business school and was now getting ready for a new job far from home. "We didn't ever think we'd see the day when she'd leave home," my friend said, adding, "My sister was concerned for years about her—she seemed so high strung and skittish most of the time. Frankly, I was surprised she went away to college."

Laura's Story

Laura's story started out innocently enough. When she was fourteen, she took her beloved English spaniel, Gus, for a walk. She tied Gus's leash to a parking meter while she went into a store to get a package of mints. When she came out, Laura saw that the dog had slipped its collar and was nowhere to be found. She scoured the neighborhood, checking every store, and after two traumatic days of posting fliers and soliciting help from friends, was relieved when a stranger found the dog and returned him. Stress resolved; crisis averted.

Three years later, however, when Laura was seventeen, her best friend was killed in a skiing accident. She was as devastated—emotionally and physiologically—as she'd been when she thought her dog was lost to her forever. Even more so. And this time, because her friend was not miraculously brought back (as her dog had been), her anxiety persisted as her body continued to churn out stress hormones. Eventually, she had difficulty sleeping, lost her appetite, and had problems concentrating at school. Four months later she had lost ten pounds, still wasn't sleeping well, and found it harder and harder to get out of bed in the morning.

When she left for college the following year the separation triggered a similar biological stress response. Though leaving home was far from a tragedy, it felt like a crisis to Laura, and her eating and sleeping problems started up all over again. Every time she got her period she would go into a funk, miss class, and feel despondent. With stress layering upon stress, Laura soon found herself reliving the dramatic impact of each incident until she finally crossed the line from chronic stress to SuperStress. Her brain had learned to default to crisis mode even when there was no crisis.

The fact that Laura eventually came around successfully demonstrates that even though you may currently be suffering from SuperStress, there's no reason that it must persist. *A brain that has learned to default to an agitated state can unlearn it just as easily.*

FOUR HALLMARKS OF SUPERSTRESS

Here are four hallmarks that illustrate how SuperStress differs from chronic stress. Although Laura's experience touches on all of them, you don't have to have more than one to be SuperStressed.

Stress is compounded. With chronic stress you may experience a stress-provoking situation over a period of time, maybe even two such experiences at a time, but it's not until you have a cluster of symptoms that you reach the proverbial tipping point and slide over to SuperStress.

You can't get a handle on it anymore. With chronic stress, you can have one symptom or more—including memory loss, persistent insomnia, fatigue, anxiety, or depression. But because they're compartmentalized, you can deal with each and with some work get those issues under control. It's SuperStress when you no longer feel that you can separate those symptoms. When the strain of dealing with them colors every moment of your day, when the life you're living is out of control, it's SuperStress.

Life has lost its luster. You've lost your sense of humor and your motivation. With chronic stress, you may feel this way some of the time, but with SuperStress, you feel like this more often than not. Sure, you can numb yourself by eating a hot fudge sundae, watching TV, taking a pill to go to sleep, or extending happy hour well into the night. But when you finish self-medicating your stress is right there waiting for you.

Anxious is the new normal. On a physical level, SuperStress is waking up and feeling exhausted, as if your body is desperately fighting off an attack from an enemy that never lets up. Your default mental state is a state of depression, anxiety, or apathy. You simply don't feel *safe*. In that way, SuperStress is very much like post-traumatic stress, the condition that plagues soldiers who manage to survive life and death encounters on the front and come home to later pay the price.

TIPPING POINTS: FACTORS THAT SLIDE US INTO SUPERSTRESS

Although everyone's response to stress is different, certain factors are universal in the ways that influence how stress affects us all. Your age, personality, gender, and genetic makeup can all have a bearing on how you respond to stressors. So can the broader context of your life, such as your support systems, social skills, and relationships. Your self-esteem is important, as are your coping mechanisms and what you do for a living. Spiritual factors play a role, and so do environmental issues such as noise pollution. Some of these things you can alter, or try to—how well you get along with your mother-in-law, for example. But your genetics or the circumstances that you experienced in childhood are not as mutable—they'll always be a part of who you are. With motivation and the proper attention, issues related to uncontrollable stress factors can easily be resolved.

Friends and Family

Whoever said "a problem shared is a problem halved" knew of what they spoke. Living in isolation, without the support of family or friends, not only increases allostatic load; it's a superhighway to Super-Stress. We all need a supportive person or two with whom we can share our good times and bad times. People need *people*. Being able to ventilate, cry, or just have someone listen to you is often enough to help you put a very stressful situation into perspective. In fact, most scientific studies cite social support as the number one determinant of how people handle a stressful situation. Walk into any surgical waiting room and you'll probably find several "waiters" for every patient being operated on. Belonging to a community—whether it's a knitting circle, a sports league, cat fancier's club, or a monthly dinner group with friends—is an important component of the Four-Week Solution you'll find later in the book. It's a known fact that the brain cannot process two opposite feelings at the same time. Think about it: you can't be both happy and unhappy. So, if you're in the company of friends and loved ones, you may have stress, but it's guaranteed to diminish by leaps and bounds from what you might feel in isolation.

Status Matters

Where you fall on the social scale plays a large role in how you feel about yourself. This isn't news. Although I should amend that sentence to read, Your place on the social scale *can* play a large role. Not everyone is hung up on who has what and who has more. But many of us are. The underpinning of capitalism is no longer keeping up with the Joneses, but *surpassing* the Joneses. Does money buy status? Maybe. But we know it doesn't buy happiness. A slew of scientific studies tell us that lottery winners are happy for a short period of time and then go back to their prewinning state of contentment—or discontentment. We're all imprinted in some way with *wanton wanting*. Enough is never enough. You know the litany: a guy builds his million-dollar dream house and six months later his next-door neighbor puts up a two-million-dollar one. Is the guy in the first house happy? What do you think?

Two interesting studies, led by Dr. Nancy E. Adler of the University of California at San Francisco, reinforce the connection between status and stress, demonstrating that our well-being—not just our happiness—is profoundly affected by our social status. The first shows how income and education are as important to our health as is our *perception* of our social status.[2] The second found that women who ranked themselves higher on the social ladder reported better physical health, had lower resting cortisol levels (a stress barometer), and less abdominal fat than women who placed themselves on lower rungs.[3] Abdominal fat is inextricably, maddeningly linked to the hormone cortisol, and to stress.

Day-to-Day Hassles

Hassles equal stress. More hassles equal more stress. By now, you know this. And I certainly know this. Let me explain that last sentence by citing an experience that I had in the last twenty-four hours during which the magnitude of the stress I felt defied all description. But I'll try anyway: I was midway through composing a paper for a scientific journal when the document on my computer went dark and a message appeared telling me that the program was forced to shut down. Oh, and by the way, the message also informed me that *my document could not be saved.* I felt as if my oxygen had been cut off. But I decided in the interest of this book to moderate my stress response. And so I began to breathe in and count to four, breathe out and count to four, breathe in . . . and so on for five minutes. And then I picked up the phone. My first call was to the big box store where I purchased the computer less than a year ago. After listening to no less than five disembodied voices informing me which numbers to press for which department, I finally got to speak to a person who told me—can you guess?—to contact the manufacturer of the computer! I did. And lo and behold, ten minutes later someone in Bangalore was asking me a battery of questions which I did the best I could to answer, and I was eventually connected to technical support.

I'll spare you the details other than to say that two hours and several disconnects, redials, and breathing exercises later, my computer actually got up and running again. (And yes, my document had even been saved!) The moral of the story? It doesn't matter if you're reading a book or writing one, or how much you think you're exempt, if you live in today's world and are the proud owner of all of today's stuff, sooner or later stress is going to get you. The goal is to know how to handle it when it does.

Parenting—and "Childing"

Our parents and certainly our grandparents probably wouldn't recognize what we call parenting as anything they'd ever done—that's how all-encompassing the job has become. And I use the word *job* with great advisement. There is no limit to the number of articles, speeches, and lectures that have demonstrated the repercussions—both physical and mental—of this generation's attempts to be both superprofessionals and superparents. It's the perfect setup for SuperStress, because it's like stepping on the gas and the brake at the same time. The truth is that those two goals are mutually exclusive. Which is not to say that stay-at-home parents are immune from SuperStress; they most definitely are not. Whether we're in the office or on the playground, we all try to do the best we can for our kids, striving to give them every advantage they need to grow into us—only better. Let's face it: parenting is a competitive sport where overachieving parents see their children as achievements. If that doesn't spell SuperStress, nothing does. But let's look at the flip side.

Being a kid can be pretty stressful, too.

From early age, children are acquainted with the notion that they're competing against others for a few cherished spots in the right nursery school. By the time these children hit high school they're veterans of the high-achievement treadmill. And it's not over. With colleges so hard to get into these days, students feel that they have no choice but to take college-level courses, master an instrument, play sports, run for student council, and work on the yearbook. By the time the admission (or rejection) letters arrive, these kids are so burned out, it's a wonder that they've got anything left for college.

Job Stress

According to the American Psychological Association (APA) 2007 Stress in America survey, job stress is far and away the leading source of stress for adults. More than half of all employees interviewed (52 percent) reported that workplace stress influenced important career decisions. Because of stress-related factors, 18 percent left a job, 41 percent considered seeking a new job, and 22 percent declined a promotion.

Is there no justice? First we do everything we can to secure that demanding job and then it eats us alive. Workaholism and overstimulation are so prevalent that I'm seeing more and more patients with the same complaints. One of my newer patients, whom I'll call Sara, is a thirty-year-old woman a year out of business school. She typifies so many of the new hires in just about every major city in the developed world.

Sara's Story

On a bleak day in June, Sara came into my office drenched from the rain, hair askew. I asked her why she had come to see me.

"Oh, its just a minor problem," she said, almost apologetically, "but it's interfering with my work so I decided to fix it." (You'll notice that she wanted to fix the problem, not herself.) She told me she had landed the perfect job with a top investment-banking firm on Wall Street. "All that hard work to get into the right college and the right business school finally paid off," she said, almost forcing a smile. But she looked far from thrilled. In fact, she looked plain old tired to me. And to the point: her complaint was insomnia and the ensuing lack of energy she experienced during the day. I took her medical history, examined her, and found her to be in good health.

When we returned to my office, I asked what she did when she wasn't working.

"Oh, I try to get to bed as early as I can—given some of the crazy hours they expect of us. But that's the problem. I just can't fall asleep and if I can, I don't stay asleep very long." As she spoke, her eyes were on me, but I couldn't help notice that her hand was fishing around in her handbag. Eventually, she extracted her BlackBerry and without missing a beat, stole a glance at it. I indicated the machine and asked her about her "relationship" with it. "Well," she explained, "we're kind of tight." Another half smile. "I keep it next to my bed at night just in case, and of course during the day I'll check it every so often."

She was far from alone in her relationship with her BlackBerry. Research in Motion, the maker of that mobile email gadget, logged 6.2 million subscribers at the end of the first half of 2006, up from 3.6 million in the same period the year before.[4]

"How often would that be?" I asked her.

"Well, a few times an hour." Pause. "Okay, okay, maybe five or six."

"And at night?"

"At night, I'm up anyway, so I check my email and then I try to get back to everybody because I know I won't have time to do it during the day."

"And your weekends? What are they like?"

"Oh," she said proudly. "I don't go into the office, but I do work from home." She logged sixty to seventy hours a week at her office and spoke of it as if she had bragging rights. And she wasn't physically at her office on the weekends, but she was virtually there. Seven days a week. No wonder she was tired.

If Sara's SuperStress had become too overwhelming, she could always, in the interest of her own health, downsize her life—that is, she could resign her job and do something less stressful for a while. (Not all of us have that choice; for most of us, that's a completely unrealistic resolution.)

Instead of downsizing, for therapy, we started off with some vitamins—which you will read about in more detail later in the book. More important, I recommended several lifestyle changes, too. We structured a sleep program for her, and I gave her some meditation exercises. Then I had an idea that I knew would surely cap it off. I suggested that each evening when she returned home from work and emptied her mailbox, she store her BlackBerry there overnight. (Yes, in the mailbox!) At first, she couldn't believe I was serious, but eventually we made a compromise—she'd lock up her BlackBerry two nights a week for starters and see what happened. In case you're wondering, like I was, if such an experiment could possibly work, it did. And it didn't. She was successful for the first week, but it was, as she later told me, like stopping smoking cold turkey with the aftereffect of a caffeine headache. Well, not really that bad, but it wasn't pleasant. She was mostly bored. But she became aware of her BlackBerry dependence, and has since resolved to pay closer attention to how often she uses the device.

UNCONTROLLABLE STRESS FACTORS

There are some things we can only react *to* (rather than control) and these include our heredity and our early childhood experiences, both of which play extremely important roles in determining our vulnerability to SuperStress.

Genetic predisposition and early developmental events influence the ways in which we respond to certain occurrences throughout our lives. Severe stress in early life seems to play a key role in why some adults appear more vulnerable than others to stressful situations. Several studies bear this out. One study led by Dr. Charles Nemeroff, a psychiatrist at Emory University, found that women who were sexually or physically abused as children secreted more stress hormones when faced with even the mildest of stressful situations than women who never experienced abuse in childhood.[5] In an animal study published by Dr. Michael Meaney, PhD in the departments of psychiatry and neurology at McGill University, rat pups were removed from their mothers for ten-minute intervals.[6] The mothers, so happy to see the pups returned, showered them with attention above and beyond what they might have had in normal circumstances. The findings showed that as the babies became older, they were more confident and secreted lower levels of the stress hormone in stressful situations than did rats who had lacked such attention. This effect lasted for the animal's lifetime.

HORMONES: THE OIL THAT GREASES THE WHEELS OF STRESS

Hormones are the chemical messengers that our bodies produce and release in order to trigger a wide variety of processes. They help regulate our blood sugar and insulin levels as well as our growth. Cortisol and epinephrine are the two hormones primarily responsible for the stress response in both males and females. These are not, however, the only hormones that affect the stress response. Estrogen, progesterone, testosterone, and oxytocin are also involved, although they might be said to have supporting roles. This is where the gender issue slowly creeps into play. Let's take a closer look at how a man's and a woman's hormones are affected by, and in turn affect, SuperStress.

Cortisol: Good Cop / Bad Cop

The stressors that our ancestors encountered—starvation, injury, freezing weather—were physical. To cope with these emergencies, cortisol broke down nonessential organs and tissues in order to maintain blood sugar levels and bring life-enhancing nutrients to the vital organs. In those days, cortisol was a "good cop," directing lifesaving resources to help the body fight the attacker. Today's stressors, however—a bad marriage, financial problems—tend to be chronic and psychological, rather than physical. Remember, our brains do not know the difference, so they respond in the way they always have—by secreting more cortisol. But cortisol, under chronic exposure, is a "bad cop," whose "the more the better" approach can destroy healthy muscle and bone; delay healing and normal cell regeneration; impair digestion, metabolism, and mental function; and weaken your immune system. High levels of cortisol also produce elevated blood fats and sugar, which are related to many disorders, including diabetes, heart disease, and inflammation.

In a SuperStress situation, women will always generate more cortisol than men because in the second half of the menstrual cycle, women produce progesterone, which keeps cortisol surging even after the stress response is over. In other words, women are more likely than men to have their stress circuits get stuck in the "on" position, which would explain why the ratio of women to men who report suffering stress may be as high as 3:1.

Cortisol is a bane to women in other ways, too. For starters, research has shown that cortisol not only stimulates the appetite, but also specifically induces cravings for sugar and fat. It's the devil on our shoulder that urges us to eat when we're stressed, and to reach for the leftover banana cream pie rather than any of those fresh vegetables you brought back from the farmers' market. And there's more bad news: once you've consumed all that fat, cortisol instructs your body to store it—and even tells you *where* to store it. Any guesses? Yes, that fat is routed on an express track to your belly! That's nature's way of insuring that there will be fuel at the ready in case of a famine. But nature didn't count on an extended feast. This issue is far more important than battling with the top button of last summer's skinny jeans. Fat on the belly is no laughing matter. It can, in fact, kill you.

THERE ARE TWO TYPES OF BELLY FAT: *subcutaneous* and *visceral.* Because one of them is so closely related to SuperStress, and so potentially dangerous, it's essential to be able to distinguish between the two. Subcutaneous (under the skin) belly fat sits atop your abdominal muscles, jiggles when you walk, and is the reason sweats become the outfit of choice whenever possible. While subcutaneous fat can be annoying, it's not nearly as threatening to your health as the second type, visceral fat, too much of which can actually be deadly.

Visceral fat lies deep within the body cavity, beneath the abdominal muscles. Visceral fat surrounds the vital organs, including the heart, kidneys, and liver—and it's impossible to detect without an MRI. Scientists once believed that fat cells did nothing more than shrink and grow, depending on what you had for dinner. Today we know that fat is alive and active and busy secreting its own set of hormones. Which brings us back to cortisol and the most vicious of cycles: Stress encourages the release of cortisol. SuperStress creates super amounts of cortisol. Cortisol targets visceral fat cells, encouraging the creation of more visceral fat and opening you up to any number of serious diseases.

If you're wondering about your own belly fat, you can easily measure whether or not you have a reason for concern. The National Institutes of Health tell us that the best way to determine if you're healthy is not to hop on the scale, but to pull out the tape measure. The widest part of the belly should measure no larger than thirty-five inches in a woman and forty inches in a man. *Anything above that becomes dangerous to your health.*

Love Is . . . Oxytocin

Fortunately, nature designed a built-in mechanism for moderating stress that involves oxytocin. If you are a woman and have children, you may remember reading in one of the pregnancy guides you bought that oxytocin induces emotional bonding as well as labor and lactation. Here's the good news: oxytocin also directly counters the effects of cortisol. While cortisol is the hormone of fear, oxytocin is the hormone of love. If cortisol brings feelings of aggression, anxiety, and hyperactivity, oxytocin fosters positive feelings of calmness and connection. Cortisol suppresses libido; oxytocin increases sexual receptivity. And while cortisol breaks down muscles, bones, and joints, oxytocin repairs and restores them. It's the heart's friend, too, because while cortisol increases blood pressure, oxytocin lowers it.

Though you won't find it on the grocery store's shelves, oxytocin is far from out of reach. Meditation, yoga, exercise, massage, caring for a pet, and joining a support group all promote this warm fuzzy hormone's production, as do intimate relationships. Oxytocin is the biochemical manifestation of love. We produce it when we love and are loved, give of ourselves, or engage in the warmth of bonding.

Estrogen

There is no question that estrogen plays a role in protecting women against certain diseases. Cardiovascular disease (CVD) is a perfect example. Coronary artery disease is far more prevalent in men than in women, but only until such time as women hit menopause, which is when their bodies begin producing less estrogen, thus putting them on a closer hormonal level with men. Postmenopausal women suffer from as many cardiovascular ailments as men their age. In fact, CVD is the leading cause of death in women today. Prior to menopause, estrogen protects women's blood vessels by keeping them elastic, which lets them expand to allow for good blood flow. Estrogen also prevents cholesterol accumulation on the inside of blood vessels. So, when the estrogen diminishes in a woman's body, so do its benefits.

But an animal study done at Yale University showed that estrogen amplified the stress response in the areas of the brain that are most closely related to depression and other stress-related illnesses.[7] Rebecca Shansky, the Yale team leader, exposed both male and female rats to different levels of mild stress and then tested them with short-term memory tasks. The study found that males and females performed equally well on the tasks while under mild stress and in the absence of stress, and both performed poorly when exposed to high levels of stress. The difference was that when female rats were in a high-estrogen phase, they were more sensitive to the effects of stress: they perceived more stress and performed worse. To establish that estrogen really was the cause of this difference, Shansky next removed the ovaries of a new group of females, thereby stripping them of any natural estrogen they might have produced. She split the group into two and planted a time-release capsule containing estrogen in one group and a placebo in the other. When she repeated the experiment the animals with the placebo showed no effects, while the animals given estrogen replacement had the same results as the animals with natural estrogen. She had found the culprit—estrogen did enhance the stress response and cause greater stress-related impairments.

Over time, women generate more cortisol than men because in the second half of the menstrual cycle they produce progesterone, a hormone that ensures ongoing cortisol production. Consequently, as we saw earlier in this chapter, the ratio of women to men who report suffering stress may be as high as 3:1. Recent research suggests that twice as many women as men suffer from depression. Unfortunately, what evolved as a useful physical adaptation in females—encouraging them to protect their young through heightened vigilance, multitasking, and future-oriented thinking—has become a liability in the twenty-first century.

Jeannie's Story

One of my patients, Jeannie, had an especially marked hormonal response to stress. Jeannie was referred to me because of classic perimenopausal symptoms: irregular periods, "brain fog" (her term), forgetfulness, night sweats, and hot flashes. "I don't want to take hormone replacement," she said, "because I've read too many reports linking it to cancer. And I still get my period sometimes." She led what she called a "mid-coastal life," traveling twice a month from Boulder, Colorado, where she lived with her husband and children, to New York for her job. "I think it's the travel that's getting to me," she said. "I never have hot flashes or night sweats in Colorado, but in New York, exactly when I need to be in top form, they torment me."

Like most women, Jeannie carried some familiar emotional baggage. She was expected to be the ultimate career woman in New York, even though it was where she suffered from the strain of separation from her family. Stress was clearly triggering her symptoms. Most women are raised to be social facilitators and "pleasers." As a result, they feel pressure to be perfect—perfect wives, perfect mothers, and model employees. Like Jeannie, they can be wracked with doubts about their adequacy. Women are also conditioned to keep negative emotions, especially anger, to themselves.

I told Jeannie that what I thought she needed to ease her symptoms was a relaxation program that would help her nervous system remember the physiological responses that create the hormones that reverse stress. The connection between women in perimenopause and the stress response falls in the area of the adrenal glands, which also serve as a reservoir for a small amount of estrogen in perimenopausal women. To treat her hot flashes and to help her sleep better, I prescribed some herbs that work on moderating those issues. (We'll get to this in Chapter 10). After four weeks, Jeannie was doing well. Her hot flashes had abated to the point where she was comfortable, and she generally reported feeling better both at home and while on the road.

Testosterone

Stress has some positive aspects for men. In its early stages, it actually boosts mental capacity to a greater degree than it does for women. The reason for this is that the hormone testosterone blocks the release of cortisol for a short amount of time. But on the downside, men produce as much as 52 percent more serotonin, a mood-regulating neurotransmitter, than women do. This can block their awareness of stress, so when men get SuperStressed, they tend to recognize it later than women—often after the physical damage has already begun. But on the plus side, men don't retain a visceral memory of stressors, a difference probably rooted in evolution. Historically, men have been protectors, bravely taking on all comers; if they recalled in vivid detail each of the difficulties they faced while on the hunt, they might not be so willing to return to the savanna so fast.

The oxytocin story differs in men and women, too. It used to be thought that women produced more oxytocin than men, but we now know that's not true. The amount is the same, but oxytocin's effects are more limited in men because testosterone counteracts it. While oxytocin is the balm that quiets stress in women, building up testosterone is what enables stress recovery in men. When men consistently live with lower testosterone levels, prolonged interactions with people drain them. This is especially true if they lack sufficient alone time. When women and men make love, oxytocin production increases for both of them, but in men, testosterone also increases, negating some of oxytocin's benefits. So the old cliché has a very real biological source. After a couple makes love, her hormonal cocktail has her primed for cuddling while his newly elevated testosterone drops his oxytocin level, making him less interested in prolonged physical intimacy. Rather, it has him reaching for the TV remote.

Roger's Story

Roger's wife insisted he see me because, as he said, "she thinks I'm losing it." A top talent agent who, at forty-five, owns a twenty-person firm, Roger led a hectic life, constantly crisscrossing the country to serve clients or to drum up business. Even in transit, he was closing deals via BlackBerry and cell phone, fueled by caffeine in whatever form was readily at hand. He had thrived on the excitement of this lifestyle for fifteen years. But once he hit forty, his nerves seemed to unravel. He started losing his temper during negotiations and with his employees. One day he shouted at an office temp who promptly burst into tears. He felt terrible. "But," he hastened to explain, "I can't run a business with people I can't count on. I work hard and need them to work hard, too."

Roger had always thought of his employees as a second family, but now he wondered what they thought of him—was he a father figure or just a hothead? Worse yet, in recent years, his irritability had leaked outside the professional sphere. Once he was barred from boarding a flight because he'd bullied a gate attendant; stuck in traffic, he railed at cab drivers; and, out to eat with his family, he ruined meals by bellowing at his kids for minor infractions. Roger rejected the idea of psychotherapy but reported, "My wife says she's sick of living with a rageaholic. She wants me to get some supplements to calm me down." When I tried to talk to him about relaxation, he brushed the advice off with an all-too-common male response: "My business is ultra-competitive. If I snooze, I lose. I have to stay in high gear."

In the spirit of using an integrative approach, I enacted some changes for Roger in the mind/body/spirit realm. The first thing I prescribed was a weeklong vacation with his wife, leaving the kids and his BlackBerry at home. During that week, I urged him to do nothing but calming and breathing exercises for ten minutes of every hour. The idea was for him to develop the habit of building small still points into his day—times during which he could actively relax and recover. Because Roger found it hard to cultivate stillness, when he returned from vacation I hooked him up to a heart-rate variability monitor, an ingenious contraption that translates heart rate into colors along a spectrum: green and blue denote a relaxed heart rate; red denotes an elevated (stressed) heart rate or distracted mood. I asked Roger to focus on pushing the light toward the relaxing blue and green zones. After a few tries, he understood on a visceral level what he needed to do. To imprint the feeling in his body, I encouraged him to practice pushing the machine into the blue or green zone for ten minutes, twice a day. I also prescribed acupuncture to soothe his nerves and some supplements that I thought would be helpful. A month later, when he returned for a follow-up visit, he told me that he'd continued with the supplements, heart-rate variability monitor, and weekly acupuncture, and that the program was helping. He even asked me for some new relaxation techniques. Best of all, he said that reclaiming his life from SuperStress hadn't dulled his competitive edge at all. In fact, he felt more productive and energetic than he had in years.

THE PHYSICAL EFFECTS OF SUPERSTRESS

Of all the ways that SuperStress manifests, it's the physical effects that are least apparent to those who are suffering from it. But since hormones mediate moods and are the body's chemical messengers, virtually every organ from the brain to the heart to the digestive system is affected.

The Cardiovascular System

Stress affects the heart in many ways. To begin with, the surge of the stress hormones cortisol and adrenaline increase pumping action and heart rate, and also cause the blood vessels to constrict. Constricted vessels mean that the blood has a harder time returning to the heart. But the heart, because it's a muscle, requires oxygen-rich blood to maintain its pumping, and so it has to work harder to do its job. Next, stress hormones command your body fat to give up fatty acids, which ensures energy for rapid response. But fatty acids circulating in the blood quickly become cholesterol and you know that's not heart-friendly. Finally, we've seen how stress elevates blood pressure; when that goes on too long, plaque builds up in the arteries. Enough plaque buildup, and a heart attack is only a beat away.

The Brain

We learn from supercharged memories to remain alert and avoid situations that aren't good for us. The amygdala, a small almond-shaped section of the brain, remembers mostly emotionally charged positive or negative events. It stores memories of anything that frightened us in the past, even things we wish we could forget. It is why we automatically avoid touching the base of an iron to see if it's on—having once been burned. It's also why a Vietnam veteran can be playing golf thirty-five years after the war when, hearing the *pop* of a golf cart backfiring, he "hits the deck" exactly as he did when he was running from sniper fire in the jungle. The amygdala alerts us to what it recognizes as danger—even when it's cued by something that is not really dangerous.

But, as with the heart, cumulative effects of repeated stress do no good to our brains. The hormone cortisol is the culprit here, too. In the short term, cortisol can help us out of some hairy situations, but a sustained course of the hormone is not what the doctor ordered for the brain. It attacks nerve cells, neurons, in the hippocampus—the center for memory and learning—and ultimately shrinks and even kills some of them. Those that remain have fewer points of connection to other nerve cells. The setup looks like a long chain of barbells: a neuron (nerve cell) on each end connected by a synapse, and so on. Nerve cells in the brain talk to each other through these synapses in order to process information; as in the world of networking, it's all about connections. Without good ones, you're lost and so are your nerve cells. In response to stress, the webbings between brain cells that hold our most precious memories can become disconnected. Here's more: the brain is plastic—that is, it is continually regenerating itself by growing new neurons. This allows us to process new information. But it appears that repeated stress suppresses the production of *new* nerve cells, and as a result, the hippocampus itself becomes smaller, and that affects our learning capacity.

Cortisol plays a role in retrieving long- and short-term memories. Example: your husband and five children are waiting in the car to go to the zoo and you have misplaced the car keys. "Where did I have them last?" You search jacket pockets, your handbag, and your diaper bag. And the longer you can't find them, the more stressed you become, and the more stressed you become, the more cortisol surges, and the more it surges, the harder it is to remember where you left them. Excessive cortisol can make it difficult to retrieve long-term memories, too, which is why people get confused in a crisis. Sometimes it doesn't even take a crisis. All it may take is a walk down Main Street with a friend, and along comes another friend you'll be required to introduce to friend number one. But what's her *name*? You're drawing a blank. How can you not remember your good friend's *name*? How? You can send your stress hormones a thank-you note for that one, too.

The Digestive System

When prehistoric lion chased prehistoric man, the former's digestive system probably ratcheted up while the latter's almost shut down—the reason being that there would be no need for it. Who has time to consider a ham sandwich when they're on the run from a ferocious carnivore? Because there's no need for the normal digestive process in acutely dangerous situations, it's better to shunt the energy elsewhere, so stress hormones inhibit digestion and increase stomach acid production. And while we know now that this doesn't directly cause stomach ulcers—the bacteria *H. pylori* has been established as the culprit there—scientists believe that the increase in stomach acids eats away at the mucous lining that protects the stomach from infection, which makes it a much more hospitable place for *H. pylori*.

How SuperStress Creates Nutritional Havoc. Prolonged stress can also irritate the large intestines, causing diarrhea or constipation, cramping, and bloating, and as a result, has been shown to exacerbate irritable bowel syndrome. If you want to grasp the physiology of what can go wrong in the GI tract of a person in a SuperStressed state—and there's a lot—you should first understand the process of digestion when it goes right. Here are the *Cliff-like Notes:*

The digestive process begins in the mouth and moves to the stomach, where digestive enzymes first break down the food into tiny particles. The food is then delivered into the small intestine, where digestive enzymes and a congregation of healthy probiotic flora are waiting. The digestive enzymes continue breaking down the food, chewing it into increasingly smaller protein, fat, and carbohydrate food molecules, readying them for release into the bloodstream through the intestinal walls. The bloodstream carries the food to cells throughout the body. Sounds pretty cut and dried, doesn't it? Normally, it is. Unfortunately, when SuperStress enters the picture, things begin to go wrong.

In addition to the flora in the intestine, serotonin receptors there receive signals from the brain on how to operate. When you are in a chronic stress situation, the brain calls for a slowdown and, as we've just seen, most of your energy is diverted away from digesting. As a result, you can either *over-* or *under-*secrete stomach acid. If you over-secrete stomach acid for any length of time, you're going to suffer from reflux or, worse still, Barret's esophagus, which is a chronic form of peptic ulcer disease that occurs as a result of longstanding reflux. The prolonged and constant exposure to a hyperacidic environment can convert normal stomach lining cells into a precancerous state requiring close medical follow-up.

Conversely, if you undersecrete acid, you will quite possibly experience a physiological cascade of unintentional happenings. If you don't secrete enough acid, your stomach doesn't release as many digestive enzymes, *which means* you don't digest your food as effectively,

   which means that downstream in your small intestine and large colon, you have gas and bloating,

      which means the food that you were supposed to digest ferments instead,

         which means, you absorb fewer micronutrients,

            which means the population of probiotic flora and bacteria that predigests your food becomes remarkably less effective because the balance of bacteria is too low to sufficiently handle the volume of food. Thus, the nutritional environment supporting the inner lining of intestinal cells deteriorates, and as a consequence loses its effectiveness as a vital barrier preventing unwanted food molecules from penetrating into the body.

There are several results of this undesirable cascade. The most important is that your body does not receive the nourishment it needs. In other words, even though you may be eating well, if your digestion is not operating at its best, you won't get the benefits (read: energy) you need from the food you're taking in. At the same time you will be more susceptible to the ravages of inflammation. Here's why: if the food you've digested leaks through the intestine in ways it's not supposed to, it's going to get picked up by the immune system. This is especially true when you have a malnourished intestinal system that displays gaps or leaks in its walls, letting food molecules into places in the body where they have never before been. When this occurs, the immune system interprets these unwanted molecules as if they were foreign bodies. In response, the immune system signals cytokines, the messengers that rally the forces. When the forces come together to attack the foreign molecules, the result is inflammation, which can manifest itself not only as food allergies and skin rashes, but do far, far more damage than that. Inflammation can wear you down on a cellular level, which ultimately leads to depletion of micronutrients as well as a lowering of overall physical resilience.

Another way SuperStress creates nutritional havoc is in how it affects your metabolism. As stress hormones sap the body of important nutrients during the fight-or-flight situation, some 1,400 chemical changes occur. Metabolism is stepped up because the body thinks you require extra energy for survival, so even if you do receive *some* nutrients, you're going to use them at an accelerated rate. You're excreting an excess of magnesium—a calming vitamin—through your kidneys. You're overutilizing your B vitamins, all of which are crucial for healthy cell development (and in some ways make us calmer.) The lack of nutritional reserves also may explain why people who are Super-Stressed often feel so tired. One final point: Stress hormones can lower levels of serotonin and oxytocin, the calming hormones. Lack of oxytocin makes us feel disconnected and lower levels of serotonin can cause carbohydrate cravings in some of us. So if you're wondering what it was that sent you tearing into the cookie jar after work today for what seemed like no apparent reason, well, now you know.

The Immune System

It's not uncommon for people to become sick when they are stressed. But it's not the stress that makes us ill. It's the fact that stress sets up other conditions in the body that make us vulnerable to getting sick. The stress hormone circuit interacts with the immune system, causing levels of important lymphocytes to drop, which makes you more vulnerable to colds, flu, fatigue, and infection. High levels of cortisol hamper disease-fighting white blood cells because the body, thinking that it's in acute stress mode, sends the immune cells elsewhere, rather than to where they're needed. At the other end of the spectrum there's also evidence that chronic stress levels can lead to a hyperactive immune system, which increases the risk of developing autoimmune diseases like lupus or multiple sclerosis. Stress is also a known factor in the flare-up of existing autoimmune disease.

Adrenal Fatigue

The basic task of your adrenal glands is to respond to stress by rushing all your body's resources into "fight or flight" mode—that is, by increasing production of adrenaline and other hormones. In addition to increasing your heart rate and blood pressure, the adrenals release your energy stores for immediate use. Normally, the adrenal glands will supply the demands and when the challenge is over, they will rest and restore themselves for the next emergency. But because we're constantly overworked, undernourished, exposed to environmental toxins, and worrying with no let-up, we are creating a continual demand on the adrenal glands. After a while the result is adrenal fatigue. Effects of adrenal fatigue can be profound, causing such symptoms as fatigue and weakness, suppression of the immune system, hormonal imbalance, skin problems, autoimmune disorders, moodiness, or depression. Adrenal fatigue may be a factor in many stress-related conditions, including fibromyalgia and chronic fatigue syndrome.

THE PSYCHOLOGICAL EFFECTS OF SUPERSTRESS

Repeated stimulation of the stress hormones lowers the level of serotonin in the body—not something we want, because serotonin is one of the primary chemicals responsible for our good moods. Without it, we are more prone to anger and aggression. Sleep habits and appetite also are affected by serotonin.

But chemicals are far from the only connections between our emotional well-being and SuperStress. SuperStress impacts our psyche by narrowing our vision. Because we're so stressed, we default into survival mode and we cease to consider that we have options and choices. Here's a hypothetical case: Say you are a single woman, newly relocated to Los Angeles, who suffers from SuperStress. You're invited to a barbecue at a friend's house and you arrive to find a yard full of people. But rather than seizing the opportunity to mingle and meet some of them, you start thinking of things you should be doing—the report that needs finishing, the closet that needs painting, the car that needs an oil change. Instead of enjoying yourself, you can't stop thinking about the time you're wasting, so you head straight for the people you already know. A quick hello, a confession that you have work to do, an air kiss good-bye to the hostess, and you're out of there. How can you have fun when you're preoccupied by everything that *isn't* where you *are*? As for the report that's waiting for you at home? It's not due for another two weeks, but you'll feel guilty about it until it's signed, sealed, and delivered. And then you'll start second-guessing everything that went into it. This is how SuperStress affects the psyche. Nothing to see. Nothing to measure. Just pure, unadulterated anxiety and an inability to enjoy yourself. In cases like these, SuperStress is a thief. It robs you of an opportunity to live life to its fullest.

But you are its accomplice because there is biology behind the psychology. Every state of mind has a physiological consequence. SuperStress is so much more complex than your garden-variety chronic stress and so much more insidious. People with SuperStress don't realize that they're stressed at all. They can experience infinite loops of anxiety or depression or isolation—and because they have accommodated these states for so long, they have no idea of what's happening in their body. Think about how it feels to have a pebble in your shoe. If you walk with it long enough you lose the awareness that it's there. Think about living next to a train track. When you first move in, the noise drives you crazy, but in time you don't notice it. It's still there, though. For those same adaptive reasons, people with SuperStress don't feel stressed. They feel numb. And that's worse.

Feeling numb is a holding pattern, but it's nothing new. I see it in my practice all the time. I saw a gentleman—an accountant in his forties—not all that long ago. He came to me because he was unable to sleep. He had a classic case of insomnia and wanted a pill, which I prescribed because I knew that it would help him. But we didn't have a conversation about *why* he wasn't sleeping because he was so rushed he didn't have time to talk—and besides, the pill was all he really came for. The pill helped, of course—he slept. But when the prescription ran out, he had to come back. Why? Because the pill was essentially a medical Band-Aid. We didn't really get to the bottom of his chronic insomnia. And now he's not sleeping, even with the pill. I knew the first time I saw him that his chronic insomnia derived from being SuperStressed. The symptoms were obvious. Even from the little conversation we did have, I noted that he was preoccupied with his job, eating poorly, and almost on the brink of divorce. He also had an elderly father who needed him. But as far as he was concerned, *he's just fine.* As long as he has a pill to get him through the night, he'll get himself through everything else. End of story.

Except that it isn't the end of the story. The real story—the *whole* story—is that there are a lot more options out there. My patient doesn't want to hear them, though. Numbing yourself with pills, liquor, or excessive amounts of food is just delaying the inevitable. The sad part, as I see it, is that people like the accountant think they'll be just fine—as long as they have that prescription, or that drink or that cookie. But that's not living. It's another clear example of getting *better* . . . but not getting *well.*

THE BEHAVIORAL EFFECTS OF SUPERSTRESS

A portrait of stress-induced behavior would be painted with a brush that has been dipped in extremes. If, for example, you're locked in a room for six weeks studying for your Law Boards, you'll rely on behaviors you think will get you through a crisis, even though you're aware that they're not doing you any good. People who are stressed out very often neglect healthy lifestyle practices. They may smoke, they may drink more than normal, and they may eat more than normal and sleep less than normal. They take on too many projects, are always in a hurry, and commit their days to so much activity that they barely have room to breathe. Because SuperStressed people always feel that they're under the gun, their behavior is generally overly reflexive and habitual. They forget that they have choices. Rather than stop to consider what they're doing—*Do I really want this third Milky Way?*—they simply indulge themselves.

Such behaviors interact and play off one another, but never with good results. Let's say that you have a new manager and the two of you can't see eye-to-eye on anything. You're worried about your job being in jeopardy, and now that your coworkers are onto the scent, they've begun to distance themselves from you. To make yourself feel better, you indulge in some retail therapy at Bloomingdale's, even though your credit card is almost maxed out from a similar binge last week. You start biting your nails again, and pretty soon you're not sleeping well, either. Sleep deprivation is known to increase appetite, so you're almost doomed to eat more. And then comes the coup de grâce. Your boyfriend calls at 11:30 at night and breaks up with you. Well, how better to get over that one than with a midnight raid on the refrigerator? And what are you going to look for when you get there?

Not a spinach salad, I can promise you that.

You're going to head for the comfort food, which will of course remind you of Mom, but it will also pile on the calories and eventually the pounds. Now you're shouldering a double whammy: you're not only back in the dating market, you're also feeling fat. At this point you may feel very alone, but you're not. In the American Psychological Association 2007 survey on Stress in America, 66 percent of people who smoke say they smoke more when they are stressed. Seventeen percent of those who drank reported that in the week prior to the study they drank too much when stressed. Half of adults (48 percent) find sleep doesn't come easily when they are stressed and nearly half (43 percent) overeat or eat unhealthy foods.

WHEN STRESS DISTURBS SLEEP

There are, of course, a number of obvious reasons we can't sleep well, many of which you've probably known about for years: drinking coffee late at night, exercising before going to bed, napping too close to bedtime, watching a horror movie from the safety of your bed. But the big-ticket item that can keep you up nights—and you surely know this from experience—is stress. And if you're in a state of SuperStress— well, it's almost a given that you're going to have chronic sleep problems.

But why do some people lose sleep during periods of stress, while others seem to be able to sleep no matter how much stress they're under? Several studies have looked at this very question. One answer might lie in the fact that different people relate to the world in different ways. Dr. Avi Sadeh of Tel Aviv University studied the sleep patterns of thirty-six students aged twenty-two to thirty-two during a routine week of studies (low stress) and again during a highly stressful month.[8] He found that those he categorized as anxious and concerned slept fewer hours in both cases than those who tended not to dwell on their emotions and could therefore shut themselves off from stress, providing more scientific proof of what we who are first-class worriers already know.

Hormones play a supporting role in the way stress affects our nightly drama. Researchers at Pennsylvania State University College of Medicine believe that they have discovered a reason why middle-aged men may lose sleep.[9] As men age, they become more sensitive to the stimulating effects of corticotropin-releasing hormone (CRH), another stress-related hormone. For the purposes of the study, both young and middle-aged men were administered CRH. The older men took longer to fall asleep and slept less deeply than the younger ones, suggesting that chronic insomnia in middle age may be the result of sensitivity to stress hormones such as CRH and cortisol.

In another study by the same group, when researchers compared patients with insomnia to those without sleep disturbances, they found that "insomniacs with the highest degree of sleep disturbance secreted the highest amount of cortisol, particularly in the evening and night-time hours." This suggests, the scientists say, that chronic insomnia is a disorder of sustained hyperarousal of the body's stress response system.[10]

HOW SLEEP DEPRIVATION AFFECTS US

Although most people tend to deny or dismiss the effects of insufficient sleep, studies of sleep-deprived people have shown that it can be serious. Those who accumulate a large sleep deficit experience attention lapses, reduced short-term memory capacity, impaired judgment, and what Dr. Stanley Coren, professor of psychology at the University of

British Columbia, refers to as "micro sleeps," which he defines as "a short period of time, usually between 10 seconds and 1 minute, in which the brain enters a sleep state regardless of what the person is doing at the time." Coren says thanks to our "high-tech, clock-driven life style," Americans now accumulate a sleep deficit that averages five hundred hours a year per person.[11]

Forget trying to store up sleep, though. Sure, an hourlong afternoon nap (am I dreaming?) would go a long way toward paying off the national sleep debt. Even fifteen or twenty minutes of sleep at midday can do much to restore alertness and efficiency. And don't forget the power nap! But sleep experts tell us that it isn't possible to bank sleep credits, even by sleeping more on weekends.

Sleep deprivation is a major concern to people with SuperStress because they don't sleep as well or as long as their nonstressed counterparts. If this describes you, you may not be relaxing, either, which is a big burden on a body that's running all the time. Without realizing it, you are quietly secreting hormones such as cortisol, which makes it difficult for the body to recuperate. The effects of long-term, cortisol-induced sleep deprivation on people who are already SuperStressed can lead to some pretty undesirable consequences.

Diminished mental performance. No less than air, water, and food, sleep is crucial to brain function. Sleep deprivation diminishes mental performance, and potentially creates brain fog, judgment lapses, and inability to store the day's activities in permanent memory.

Sleep obesity. Say it isn't so! Something else that expands the waist? How, you may be wondering, can a lack of sleep make you fat? It's evolutionary, my dear Watson. The theory is that early humans stored fat during the summer, when food was plentiful and nights were short. When we sleep for only a short period of time, our brain is fooled into thinking it's summer and signals the body to put on pounds in preparation for the long winter nights ahead. Another theory implicates two appetite-related hormones, leptin and ghrelin, as being affected by sleep deprivation. Leptin, which controls appetite, appears to fall when we have too little sleep. Ghrelin, which stimulates the appetite, rises when we sleep for too few hours. A rise in ghrelin sends the sleep-deprived right to the pantry to down just about anything that's accessible. Of course, there's always the commonsense explanation that people who can't sleep need something to do. And what's more diverting (or enjoyable) than raiding the refrigerator at three in the morning? Last up is cortisol. Prolonged sleeplessness causes the body to release cortisol into the bloodstream. Cortisol is the belly's host to belly fat. The more cortisol, the greater the invitation for fat to go directly to your midsection. But you already know that.

Type 2 diabetes. Sleeplessness puts you at risk of developing type 2 diabetes. Once more, cortisol, which regulates the blood sugar glucose, seems to be the culprit. Excessive blood sugar causes a rise in glucose in the blood that cues the body to release increasing amounts of insulin in an attempt to lower the glucose level. Over time, the process leads to insulin resistance, a condition in which the cells no longer respond to the effects of insulin. Insulin resistance can result in type 2 diabetes. Excess insulin in the blood also encourages the body to store fat, once again boosting the risk of obesity.

Early aging. Dr. Eve Van Cauter, professor of medicine at the University of Chicago, found that metabolic and hormonal changes resulting from a significant sleep debt produce results that are similar to many of the characteristics of aging. Further, Dr. Cauter says that "chronic sleep loss may not only hasten the onset but could also increase the severity of age-related ailments such as diabetes, hypertension, obesity, and memory loss."[12]

Mood shifts. In the first neural investigation into what happens to the emotional brain without sleep, results from a brain imaging study suggest that while a good night's rest can regulate your mood and help you cope with the next day's emotional challenges, sleep deprivation creates just the opposite effect by boosting the part of the brain most closely connected to depression, anxiety, and other psychiatric disorders. Matthew Walker, director of the University of California at Berkeley's Sleep and Neuroimaging Laboratory and senior author of the study, says, "It's almost as though, without sleep, the brain had reverted back to more primitive patterns of activity, in that it was unable to put emotional experiences into context and produce controlled, appropriate responses."[13]

TELOMERES AND INFLAMMATION: THE LATEST IN STRESS-RELATED SCIENCE

I would feel I was doing you a disservice if I didn't mention the latest in cutting-edge, stress-related science. So let's begin with the science behind *telomeres*—perhaps a word you have never heard before—and aging.

Telomeres

It has now been scientifically proven that psychological stress leads to premature aging and the earlier onset of diseases connected to aging. Dr. Elizabeth Blackburn and Dr. Elissa Epel, researchers at the University of California, believe that this has everything to do with the way our cells age. In a recent study, Blackburn, Epel, and their colleagues showed that chronic psychological stress—both perceived stress and real—is significantly associated with telomeres.[14] These are DNA-protein complexes that cap chromosomal ends in much the same way the plastic tip of a shoelace protects it from unraveling. Each time a cell divides, its telomere loses a small bit of DNA. When the telomere becomes too short, the cell can no longer divide. In effect, telomere shortening acts as a kind of chromosomal clock, counting down the cellular generations. Shorter telomere length is directly connected with how our cells age—and subsequently, how *we* age.

How is this all related to stress? When you have a chronic disease—including chronic stress—the telomeres shorten more quickly. What keeps them from shrinking too fast is telomerase, a repair enzyme that progressively elongates the telomeres. As we age, telomerase lessens so we don't have as much repair material roaming around our bodies. Drs. Blackburn and Epel and their colleagues have done a series of research projects based on telomeres and telomerase. In one of them, they measured at various points in time the telomeres of women who were caregivers to chronically ill patients and the telomeres of noncaregiving women, who were less stressed. The results showed that women with the highest levels of perceived stress have telomeres that are shorter on average by the equivalent of *at least one decade of additional aging* compared to the women whose stress was lower. But what was even more astonishing was that when these same caregivers were taught a stress reduction exercise, after a time their telomeres began to lengthen. This was the first time in which a mood state was both correlated with genes and shown to have a component of reversibility. These findings have strong implications for understanding how, at the cellular level, stress promotes both early aging and early onset of age-related diseases.

Inflammation

Inflammation is a physiological phenomenon that plays a big role in chronic disease and aging. If I mention arthritis as a typical disease that is associated with inflammation most people understand what I am referring to. But inflammation also has been linked to coronary artery disease, asthma, Alzheimer's, some types of cancer, and even mood states such as depression and anxiety. Although in these cases inflammation is not the only cause of the medical problem, we now know that it is a major component of how the illness is created.

Like all processes in the body, a little inflammation is useful but a lot is too much for the body to handle and thus is harmful. The state in which inflammation is positive is one in which something has changed and the inflammation alerts the body to fix it. The classic example is when you bruise yourself or have a sprain. Inflammatory cells go to the area, causing redness, heat, and swelling because of the increased circulation there. Other cells arrive, and they all begin to repair tissue. Then the inflammation goes away and you're good to go. That's the body's natural defense and it's very much like its response to acute stress—a natural and positive adaptive strategy.

What makes inflammation deadly is when, like chronic stress, it continues too long. Chronic inflammation can lead to atherosclerosis (thickening and loss of elasticity in blood vessels, causing heart disease), high blood pressure (which causes strokes), insulin resistance (which leads to diabetes), obesity, kidney failure, and such autoimmune diseases as asthma, allergies, rheumatoid arthritis, and lupus. A classic example of inflammation gone bad is coronary artery disease, which is the number-one killer of men and women. Coronary artery disease is caused by three possible components: platelet clumping, cholesterol, and inflammation. Inflammation is the part that increases the damage to the vessels of the heart. When the plaque from cholesterol imbeds into the lining of the arteries, the cytokines are signaled by the damage to come and fix it. The cells do come to repair the damage, but the problem is that once they're there, they can't escape. Eventually, the cells crowd the interior of the vessel, narrowing it like a straw that slowly clogs from the fruit in a smoothie. When the artery narrows so much that it completely closes off, a heart attack occurs.

We know from the latest research that certain states of mind are correlated with inflammation. The latest research shows that anxiety, depression, and PTSD heighten it. And because inflammation is a natural part of both aging and chronic disease, if you find yourself in a SuperStressed state you're basically pouring gasoline on a bonfire. That's because SuperStress affects so many areas of your health: you're not sleeping, your digestion isn't working, and your immune system is depressed. Add to that the fact that you're increasing inflammation, and any disease you have is going to get worse. Fortunately, the body can shut off inflammation with alternate pathways. Certain foods, botanicals, some forms of alternative therapy, and even stress reduction techniques can reduce inflammation and put out the fire.

NOT A PRETTY PICTURE, all this talk about aging and heart disease, shrunken neurons, adrenal burnout, and midnight refrigerator raids. I'm sorry to paint such an ominous portrait of what SuperStress is doing to you. But it's doing the same thing to all of us, if in different ways. The good news is that if you saw yourself in too many of the above examples and things aren't exactly as you want them to be right now, they don't have to stay that way. And if you're merely headed in the wrong direction, I can help you prevent the worst. No one has to suffer from SuperStress. *No one*. You have a choice as to how you want to live your life.

CHAPTER TWO

Assessing Your Level and Type of SuperStress

NOW THAT YOU ARE FAMILIAR with what SuperStress is and how it can manifest in the body and in one's life more generally, it's time to move on to the next step: assessing *your* level of SuperStress felt in *your* body and in *your* life. From there we will move on to the all-important issue of managing your SuperStress and your life in the best possible way.

There are plenty of books and magazine articles that will give you list upon list and tip over tip about what will work for you. But here's the problem: Do the books and magazines know you? Do they know what is causing your particular stress? Of course not. How could they, when stress manifests itself differently in each of us and, more often than not, we ourselves don't even know the cause? And how can a magazine article tell you what's best for your particular symptoms when they can't know what your symptoms are?

The SuperStress Solution program is all about *personalizing* your stress and developing personal strategies to manage it. It's about creating self-awareness so that you can understand what you need to do to have the most stress-free life possible. Fill out the following questionnaires. They won't take much time at all, but they will help you better understand what you're experiencing and determine your personal level and type of SuperStress, so that you can design your management plans.

In my experience, SuperStress symptoms appear in clusters—familiar personality and behavior patterns that correlate with specific ways in which stress is manifested. I call these clusters or patterns of behaviors "SuperStress Types." The first questionnaire identifies your SuperStress Type. There are five SuperStress personality types (see page

210 for brief descriptions of each), identifiable by the way you behave and respond to stress. Many of you, however, may see that your behavior has elements of more than one type.

The second questionnaire will show you where in your body you physically store your stress. Some people hold it all in their muscles, others in their gut; still others feel the physical repercussions of stress in their immune system.

The third questionnaire will help you identify your degree of resilience to SuperStress. The point here is to examine your lifestyle and determine if it is generally healthy—which will help you be more resilient to SuperStress—or if it could be healthier, in which case some corrections will be in order to buoy your natural resilience to stress.

The fourth questionnaire is a very quick quantification of the stressful events you have faced in the last year. Sometimes it's not until we are asked to do this kind of itemization that we gain a more clear perspective on what we've been dealing with.

The results of these questionnaires will serve as a guide for you as you proceed to Parts 2 and 3 of this book. Knowing your personal baseline—how you tend to react (your type), how stress physically affects you (where you store it), your level of resilience (or lack thereof), and the events of the last year—will determine which of the Super-Stress Solution stress-management programs is best for you. Understanding your own SuperStress profile will show you how to tailor your solution.

As you turn the page to begin these four questionnaires, remember that honesty is essential. This is private—you need not ever share the results with another soul—but it's the key to helping you find your own sanctuary.

IF YOU WOULD LIKE to take an abbreviated version of these questionnaires online, go to www.thesuperstresssolution.com.

YOUR SUPERSTRESS TYPE

How do you cope with stressful situations? How do you tend to respond under pressure? Honestly responding to the following forty questions will help you determine your SuperStress Type.

Respond to each question using the following scale:

    0 = Never
    1 = Rarely
    2 = Sometimes
    3 = Often

1. How often do others disappoint you? _____3_____
2. How often do feel close to tears? _____2_____
3. How often do you try to do everything yourself? _____3_____
4. How often do you miss the support you deserve from your coworkers? _____2_____
5. How often do you find yourself actively feuding with someone? _____2_____
6. How often do you think about personal secrets that you don't want anyone to know? _____0_____
7. How often do you have two or more major problems that you can't seem to resolve? _____2_____
8. How often do you think about people you despise? _____3_____
9. How often do you panic? _____2_____
10. How often do you feel exhausted when you wake up in the morning? _____2_____
11. How often do you yell at someone in anger? _____3_____
12. How often do you experience nervous tics, such as running your fingers through your hair, tapping your foot, licking your lips, and so on? _____2_____
13. How often do you have trouble focusing? _____3_____
14. How often do you feel stressed out? _____3_____
15. How often do you lie awake at night ruminating? _____2_____
16. How often do you feel tired during the daytime? _____3_____
17. How often do you find yourself angry with family members? _____2_____

18. How often do you feel anxious or impatient? _____

19. How often are you forgetful? _____

20. How often do you think about a beloved family member or friend who is deceased? _____

21. How often do you keep things to yourself? _____

22. How often do you feel that your life is out of control? _____

23. How often do you have difficulty sitting still? _____

24. How often do you worry about money? _____

25. How often do you cancel or put off social engagements or family outings to finish a work project? _____

26. How often do others' mannerisms annoy you? _____

27. How often do you feel as if you're going to lose control? _____

28. How often do you find yourself sensitive to criticism? _____

29. How often do you feel emotionally drained or used up at the end of the day? _____

30. How often do you view situations as win-or-lose propositions? _____

31. How often are you easily distracted? _____

32. How often do you feel lonely? _____

33. How often do you put off things till later? _____

34. How often is your stomach tied up in knots? _____

35. How often do you interrupt people when they are talking to you? _____

36. How often do you fail to see the humor in situations most people find funny? _____

37. How often are you angry with yourself? _____

38. How often do you feel that there aren't enough hours in the day to accomplish what you need to do? _____

39. How often do you worry about a terrorist attack where you live or work? _____

40. How often do you think that most people you deal with are incompetent? _____

Scoring:

Add up your scores for the following groups of questions. Write your total score in the space provided. Whichever number is the highest indicates your most frequent corresponding SuperStress Type. That said, most people who experience SuperStress will see that although they may have a high score for one type, they have an almost as high (or even equally high) score for another type. This demonstrates, of course, that SuperStress isn't an isolated phenomenon and doesn't manifest in a precise or uniform way. The important lesson here is to start paying attention to your pattern or patterns for dealing with stress.

You'll want to have this information so that you can best tailor your stress management. Starting on page 209, I'll tell you which of the stress-reduction techniques and programs are best for each type of SuperStress personality.

1. **Type I: Burned Out, Exhausted, Numb, Depressed:**
   Total the following questions: 1, 4, 10, 16, 20, 29, 32, 36 ___24___

2. **Type II: Agitated, Overwhelmed by Life:**
   Total the following questions: 7, 11, 13, 19, 22, 27, 31, 37 ___24___

3. **Type III: Emotionally Sensitive:**
   Total the following questions: 2, 9, 14, 18, 24, 28, 34, 39 ___21___

4. **Type IV: Driven, Controlling:**
   Total the following questions: 3, 6, 15, 21, 25, 30, 33, 38 ___21___

5. **Type V: Explosive, Can't Slow Down:**
   Total the following questions: 5, 8, 12, 17, 23, 26, 35, 40 ___26___

THE PHYSICAL TOLL STRESS TAKES

Respond to each question using the following scale:

0 = Never

1 = Rarely

2 = Sometimes

3 = Often

Which of the following have you experienced in the last six months?

1. Headaches _____
2. Neck aches _____
3. Backaches _____
4. Muscular tension _____
5. Bloating _____
6. Indigestion/upset stomach _____
7. Chronic constipation _____
8. Chronic diarrhea _____
9. Change in appetite _____
10. Frequent urination _____
11. Irritability _____
12. Tearfulness _____
13. Anger _____
14. Restlessness _____
15. Frequent illness _____
16. Insomnia _____
17. Fatigue _____
18. Faintness or dizziness _____
19. Heart palpitations _____
20. Cold hands and feet _____
21. Hot flashes _____
22. Trouble concentrating _____
23. Loss of sex drive _____
24. Loss of stamina _____

A. Total the following questions:

1, 2, 3, 4 _____12_____

B. Total the following questions:

5, 6, 7, 8, 9, 10, 23 ___21_____

C. Total the following questions:

11, 12, 13, 14, 15, 16, 17 __21_____

D. Total the following questions:

18, 19, 20, 21, 22, 24 ___21_____

A. Reflects the degree of SuperStress in the musculoskeletal system

B. Reflects the degree of SuperStress in the gastrointestinal and urinary system

C. Reflects the degree of SuperStress as a psychological disturbance

D. Reflects the degree of SuperStress overtaxing your adrenal (energy) system

The higher your score, the greater the pressure on that system from SuperStress. Your stress may show up in one, two, three, or even all four categories. Once you see where the symptoms of your stress are greatest, you can treat the symptoms by going to Chapter 10, where you will find the specific integrative therapies for each situation. Now, it's possible that you may not find your symptoms listed here because there just wasn't room to list every stress-associated difficulty. But if you are experiencing such ailments as loss of hair, dry skin and nails, forgetfulness, even worsening of PMS symptoms, write these symptoms on the right-hand side of your test so you can see the additional ways *you* express stress in your body. And though the exact solution may not be explicitly spelled out herein, my suggestion is to use the four-week plan and track its effectiveness at improving your own stress-related symptoms.

Note: If you are experiencing any of these symptoms chronically, it is wise to have a medical evaluation.

QUESTIONNAIRE #3
YOUR PERSONAL RESILIENCE TO SUPERSTRESS

This questionnaire is designed to uncover lifestyle issues that may be caused by or result in SuperStress. The higher your scores for each, the lower your resilience and the harder it will be to bounce back from stress.

Respond to each question using the following scale:

   0 = Never
   1 = Rarely
   2 = Sometimes
   3 = Often

1. How often do you have trouble falling asleep? _____
2. How often do you sleep more than five or six consecutive hours at night? _____
3. How often do you self-medicate with drugs and/or alcohol? _____
4. How often do you eat while driving or walking? _____
5. How often do you feel like you are getting sick? _____
6. How often do you smoke? _____
7. How often during meals and meetings do you respond to emails/text messages on your PDA or cell phone? _____
8. How often does your work take you away from your family on weekends and evenings? _____
9. How often do you crave sweet/salty foods? _____
10. How often do you overeat? _____
11. How often do you think that watching TV is the most relaxing activity you do? _____
12. How often do you leave the TV on for companionship? _____
13. How often do you skip meals because you are too busy to eat? _____

   Total your answers here _____
   A score of 1–5 is a healthy amount of stress-related activity.
   A score of 6–13 indicates a modest amount of stress-related lifestyle changes.

A score of 13–25 indicates a moderate amount of stress-related lifestyle changes.

A score of 26–39 indicates an extreme or substantial amount of stress-related lifestyle changes.

If most of your answers are 0, you're a resilient person who deals directly with your problems instead of waiting for them to resolve themselves. Though you may occasionally experience SuperStress, you are probably in good enough shape to withstand many of its harmful physical effects. You may want to take a long, hard look at these issues to which you answered "sometimes" and try to modify them by paying attention to each in its own time. Mostly 3 (3 = often) answers reflect relatively poor coping mechanisms. In this case, it might be in your best interest to seek medical help so that you can begin to change the way you perceive problems. Many of the stress-reduction strategies I teach you in the following chapters will also go a long way toward alleviating the stress you feel from these events.

QUESTIONNAIRE #4
RECENT STRESSFUL EVENTS

The questionnaire below is designed to help build your awareness of the stressful events you have faced recently. In a SuperStress environment, one of the first things we lose is perspective. This questionnaire lists the most significant positive and negative life stressors and rates whether you've experienced normal, modest, or extreme life stressors.

Check the following life changes that may have occurred in the past one to two years.

EVENTS OF SIGNIFICANCE	YES	NO
1. Move to a new home		
2. Death of a family member or close friend *		
3. Loss of a job *		
4. Divorce or breakup of a significant relationship*		
5. Failure of an important project		
6. Significant change in financial status (good or bad)		
7. Major change in work schedule		
8. Birth of a child		
9. Child left home for college		
10. Child got married		
11. Married or moved in with significant other		
12. Health problems (self or someone close)		
13. Threatened eviction or foreclosure *		
14. Caretaker role*		
15. Trouble with a boss/superior		

If something comes to mind that is not on the list that represents a stressor, write it down here and rate it from 1–10. You don't need to add it to the score below but rating it for yourself will give you insight on how much it may be weighing on you without your awareness. _____

Score one point for each yes answer except those followed by an asterisk (*). Those yes asterisk answers should be assigned eleven points, because each alone is a source of extreme stress.

A score of 0–5 indicates normal to modest life stress.

A score of 6–10 indicates moderate life stress.

A score of 11 or higher indicates that you have had extreme life stress.

Place the total from the 15 questions here: _____

PUTTING IT ALL TOGETHER

My type is (place your answer from questionnaire #1) _____

Stress is stored in these systems in my body (place your answer from questionnaire #2) _____

My stress resilience score showed (place your answer from questionnaire #3)

_____

My life stress level is (place your answer from questionnaire #4)

_____

At this point, you should be well acquainted with your stress patterns. Now that you've assessed the problems, you're ready to start working on the solutions. The final two parts of this book are focused on exactly that.

PART 2

Tools for Change

NOW THAT YOU HAVE FINISHED YOUR QUESTIONNAIRES, you should have a better sense of your SuperStressed state: whether you are plagued by internal or external stressors (or both), what type of Super-Stress personality you are, and how your SuperStress has manifested physically. The tools you'll be learning about in this next section are the keys to beginning to counteract the SuperStress you have just iden-tified in yourself. You will use them over and over on your journey from a SuperStressed state to a stress-resilient one. These tools will help you change your lifestyle for the better. They are woven through-out the four-week program in the next section of this book.

Because these tools are the foundation of the program, it's essen-tial that you understand how they work and what they'll be doing for you. A short biology recap is in order. In non-SuperStressed people, the recovery response follows the stress response. As the hormones from the stress response slowly diminish in the bloodstream, the hormones orchestrated primarily by the parasympathetic nervous system—endorphins and oxytocin—replace them. Oxytocin relaxes us and cre-ates the overall sensation of well-being. Endorphins flood the body with feelings of happiness and give the all-clear signal. A body that feels safe can restore itself. A body that is relaxed also can restore itself and eventually will return to its prestressed state. This is the aim of each of the tools you will be using: to prompt your parasympathetic nervous system to secrete the hormones of serenity so that rather than feeling the unpleasant physical effects of SuperStress, you will instead feel relaxed and calm.

Because mine is an integrative approach to healing, the tools I have selected to include in the four-week program, which I will detail here in the six chapters of Part 2, involve the mind, body, and spirit.

THE PATHWAYS TO PEACE describes exercises that fall within the realm of mindfulness. They may not seem like they are doing much for SuperStress but believe me, they are.

FOODS THAT HEAL. There are foods, and there are *foods*! The ones we're interested in are the ones that can actually improve our resistance to the damaging effects of SuperStress.

REST AND MOTION. In this chapter you'll learn ways to step up your physical activity as well as tips for better sleep and relaxation techniques, both of which will supercharge your recovery processes.

MIND OVER SUPERSTRESS. Research has shown that if you're an optimist who always sees the brighter side of things, you probably feel that you experience more positive events in your life than others, find yourself less stressed, and even enjoy greater health benefits. If you aren't one of those people, this chapter will help you move in that direction.

THE POWER OF CONNECTION. Our association with our immediate and larger communities is an essential part of a healthy lifestyle. We'll talk here about the benefits of belonging to a social group and volunteering, which can offer the deep satisfaction that comes with giving back.

THE LIFE OF THE SPIRIT. SuperStress sufferers are often in a state of spiritual crisis. They are so focused on merely getting through each day that they lose their grip on healthy values, such as empathy and compassion. Embracing your spirituality will help you manage difficult times.

WHY PROCESS BEATS PILLS

If you're anything like a fairly large percentage of the people I see in my practice, you may be wondering why you need all this. Why can't you just take a few pills to drown your stress? In fact, you can. I'm a great advocate of choice, so if you choose to take Xanax or have a margarita or steep yourself in a few hours of your favorite sitcom reruns to blunt the effects of a long day, go for it. Indeed, these self-numbing measures probably *will* make you feel better. But before you indulge, understand that *you are only numbing yourself for as long as that sitcom lasts.* Where are you going to be when the Xanax wears off? Still Super-Stressed! When you come down from your margarita high, your Super-Stress will still be perched right there on your shoulder. So yes, you can choose to employ any of these measures. But they won't heal your Super-Stress. They're truly just delaying the time when you have to face it.

THE TAO OF CHANGE

As a physician, I'm always happy when people get better, but that's not my ultimate goal. My ultimate goal is for my patients to thrive, to have control over the choices they make, and to feel they're strong enough to handle most difficulties that life throws their way. This is the foundation of the gift I am giving to you with these tools and with the combination of them laid out in the four-week program: the opportunity to find peace, serenity, and an inner sanctuary when you need it. In other words, an opportunity to *thrive.* But we all know there's no free lunch. And so, I'm going to ask something of you in return: a promise that you will do your best to honor the following four-part commitment to yourself.

1. **Choose to change.**
   If you've come this far, I'm guessing you're ready to change the ways you respond to life's stressors. Fortunately, you have not one, but two opportunities to do so. You can change in an *active* way by putting the tools to work for you. When it's appropriate, you can also change the way you *perceive* the challenges you're faced with.
2. **Commit to doing what it takes to change.**
   Even though the *I Ching* (the well-known Chinese Book of Changes) tells us that change is a constant we can count on, changing one's ways is never easy. But just as you became SuperStressed through a series of small hits, you can reverse the process by taking a series of small steps toward wellness. The Japanese have a name for creating changes in small increments: They call it *Kaizen.* The Japanese believe that Kaizen is the only way to lasting change. The Lexus automobile is a great example. The makers of Toyota didn't just one day say, "Okay, let's build a car that virtually never needs repair."

They started with a model that had many flaws and kept reworking it and reworking it until one day they were able to manufacture a premier low-maintenance, high-safety automobile. In terms of our personal health, we need to do the same: change one little thing—and in a week, you'll notice a difference in the way you feel. You'll then have the courage to take the next, bigger step.

3. **Admit that you may encounter some unpleasant things along the way.**

Here is where the subconscious comes in. We like to think our choices are all conscious, rational ones. But sometimes it's our subconscious mind that's pulling the strings—and it's determined to air things we've kept buried for a long time. There's usually a reason why we blocked these things from our minds in the first place. But in order to be able to move to healthier habits, we have to bring certain things out into the light of day. The questionnaires should have started this process for you. They've helped you pinpoint the physical and emotional manifestations of the way you've been living. But now you'll have to ask yourself, How did I get to be SuperStressed? How did I end up in this terribly unhealthy position? These are questions you'll be addressing in the journaling exercise in the four-week program, and hopefully you will be able to sort out important issues and bring them to the forefront.

Sometimes revisiting the choices we've made can be painful, but there's a huge payoff. In the end you'll have a way to fight your demons—a way that doesn't require a pill or another person. You will be in control, and that is one of the great antidotes to SuperStress.

4. **Trust that you will get to a better place.**

The trust that I'm talking about is faith. Not in the religious sense, but faith in your power to rise to challenges, to overcome adversity, and to come out on the other side a little wiser and more confident that you can handle life's slings and arrows. By trusting yourself, you are giving yourself a little space to wonder what is going to happen next, knowing that if what fate deals you is not exactly what you wished for, it will be something you can manage—and that you might even learn something from the experience.

CHAPTER THREE

The Pathways to Peace

MY CLINICAL EXPERIENCE tells me that I can do more than help you alleviate SuperStress: I can guide you to a calm, centered place, where your mind, body, and spirit are in harmony. I can point you in the direction of your sanctuary, but you have to venture there yourself. This chapter illuminates the various paths that will take you there—paths that include exercises and measures recommended by traditional, conventional, and integrative practitioners. Despite their varying routes, all of these paths emerge from a single concept: that the mind and the body work best as one.

Awareness of the mind-body connection is by no means new. Until roughly three hundred years ago, virtually every medical system in the world treated the mind and the body as a single unit. This integrated approach continued in the Eastern part of the world, but by the seventeenth century, scientific and religious developments in the Western world led to what was known as a *Cartesian split*—that is, the mind and body were treated as separate and wholly distinct from each other. A few hundred years later, mind and body were reunited on the beaches of Anzio during World War II. There, with morphine for the severely wounded soldiers in dangerously short supply, Dr. Henry Beecher, a physician charged with caring for these wounded men, decided to inject them with a saline solution (water and salt), making them believe it was actually the narcotic. Despite the lack of an active ingredient, the injections seemed to help. Beecher characterized the term "placebo effect" to describe what had happened—that the mind told the body it was meant to feel less physical pain, and the body *listened*. In subsequent scientific studies Dr. Beecher showed that up to 35 percent of a therapeutic response to any medical treatment comes from the belief that you're being effectively treated—whether you actually are or not.[1]

Today, few people doubt the connection between the mind and the body. But just in case you're one of them, think back to how your heart raced the last time you misplaced your wallet.

MIND OVER MATTER— THE RELAXATION RESPONSE

Much of the credit for reuniting the mind and body belongs to Herbert Benson, M.D., a Boston cardiologist. Benson pioneered research that identified the different ways that states of mind have significant effects on the body. He showed definitively that with conscious mental effort, his subjects could induce a state of physical relaxation. Benson's claim that relaxation could be generated at will and used therapeutically for myriad physical ailments—most notably, stress—was widely heralded in medical journals and newspapers across the country, and reverence for his research continues to this day.

The seeds from which this work germinated were sown in the 1970s, when Dr. Benson began to notice that many of his cardiac patients had two risk factors in common—high blood pressure and stress. He and his colleagues at Harvard began work to test their hypothesis using monkeys as subjects. But then serendipity stepped in: a group of young practitioners of Transcendental Meditation approached him. They claimed that they were able to lower their blood pressure simply as a result of their meditation practice and asked Benson to test this hypothesis. Benson's team readily agreed. The plan was to measure the subjects' metabolism, blood pressure, heart rate, brain waves, and rate of breathing at two separate times—once when the subjects sat quietly for twenty minutes and a second time when they meditated for twenty minutes.

What the researchers were able to prove was that through the simple act of changing their thought patterns, the subjects could decrease their metabolism, breathing rate, and heart rate. They also exhibited slower brain waves, reduced oxygen consumption, and less muscular tension.

What made this discovery even more exciting was the realization that the changes were *in direct opposition to the symptoms of the stress response*. Perhaps, Benson thought, he could teach these same Transcendental Meditation methods to his patients so that, on their own, they could mentally manage the stress that was damaging them *physically*. If Dr. Benson didn't at that exact moment shout *eureka!* he should have. Because it was at that point that the "relaxation response" was born.

The relaxation response, as Benson noted, is orchestrated primarily by the parasympathetic nervous system, which puts the breaks on our stress hormones. The idea behind the relaxation response, and indeed behind each of the exercises you will find later in this chapter and again in the four-week program, is to trigger the parasympathetic nervous system to relax you, calm you, and make you feel safe so that your body can fortify itself against SuperStress. As you'll soon see, this response can be elicited by a variety of meditative techniques, including diaphragmatic breathing, repetitive prayer, tai chi, yoga, progressive muscle relaxation, and even knitting. There is also a role to be played by the integrative aspects of traditional Chinese medicine.

MEANWHILE, BACK IN THE EAST

Traditional Chinese medicine (TCM) has always integrated the body, mind, and spirit through a variety of measures such as meditation, herbal supplements, exercise, massage, and lifestyle practices. To understand the philosophy of TCM, you must first look at the three elements on which it is based—yin, yang, and qi. The traditional Chinese healer considers yin and yang to be dual and inseparable powers that regulate everything in existence. Yin represents cold, slow, or passive aspects of the person; yang represents hot, excited, or active aspects. Together they represent dark and light, motion and stillness, low and high, evil and good, disease and health, death and life. Qi represents the vital energy or life force required to regulate an individual's spiritual, emotional, mental, and physical health.

The theory underlying the practice of TCM equates good health with a true balance between yin and yang. Disease results when a disruption in the flow of qi throws off the balance of yin and yang. Taking herbs and herbal supplements, meditation, massage, and acupuncture are practices that aid healing by restoring the flow of qi and, ultimately, the yin-yang balance. The balance afforded through these practices promotes relaxation and, for people in a state of SuperStress, these measures can assist in pursuit of calm. People in a SuperStressed state never believe they're enough, and as a result, they're always trying to reach their destination but never quite get there. Eventually, they become exhausted. In the TCM philosophy, you're encouraged to think of yourself as arriving—that is, of being in a state of balance, which is the true opposite of the SuperStressed state.

A SENSORY APPROACH

In my experience, people with SuperStress are greatly helped by sensory recruitment—full engagement of the five senses. Sensory recruitment draws from life's veritable smorgasbord of pleasing sights, pleasing smells, pleasing sounds, pleasing touches—even walking in nature—and uses them as ammunition in the fight against SuperStress.

Engaging one or more of the senses in a meaningful way naturally shifts the body into parasympathetic mode, which makes your arteries relax and dilate, raises your skin temperature, and improves your digestion so that you secrete less stomach acid. Your immune system and healing powers are enhanced, and when you're sleeping, you'll secrete growth hormone. Still another benefit has to do with your blood sugar levels. Instead of spiking and plunging, your insulin levels will gradually increase and abate. All good things.

Another reason sensory recruitment is such an essential tool for the SuperStressed is because it creates an awareness of the mind and body connection. Most SuperStressed people lack such awareness; they think they're fine when they're not. They think their physical ailments—including fatigue, rashes, headaches, stomach illnesses, even colds—are rooted strictly in the body, but the symptoms are really the body's reaction to a mental stress. In the SuperStressed state, images and thoughts that exist under the surface of awareness reinforce distress.

People suffering from SuperStress have become habituated to these stimuli without even realizing that this negative circuit exists.

You may at first have a hard time believing that hypnosis, daily affirmations, or taking a walk in the woods can do much for your SuperStress. But they can. They speak a language that our conscious mind cannot always hear or understand but our limbic system (area of amygdala, hypothalamus, etc.) hears loud and clear. These tools help us feel safe and calm.

USING THE TOOLS

Read the above heading one more time! It says: *Using* the tools. It's one thing to read about these tools, and quite another to utilize them. As your stress levels rise throughout the day—and you know they will— you can employ relaxation methods to make them more manageable. As soon as you've completed one of the following exercises or undergone one of the treatments, your stress levels will once again start to climb—but each time they climb a little more slowly and take a little longer to start. In other words, your tolerance to stress builds as you manage it, until eventually you will have contained it to a level below which damaging symptoms occur. Very good news, indeed.

More important than how long you employ any of these tools is how often. Implement them regularly so that your *subconscious* mind remembers what the state of relaxation feels like. Of course I understand that you can't do all of them regularly because not all of these tools are things you can do yourself. Some, such as acupuncture and massage, are things that you need a trained therapist to employ. But for those things you can do, such as focused breathing or even yoga, know that even though the amount of time you spend at an exercise matters, it's less important than how often you do it. One recent study showed that a mere *twelve minutes* of daily meditation for eight weeks significantly increased blood flow to the brains of both normal subjects and Alzheimer's patients, greatly improving their verbal fluency, motor coordination, spatial ability, and concentration.[2] The technique used in the study is called Kirtan Kriya (see page 68), which stimulates the anterior cingulate gyrus—the area researchers believe is the optimism center in the brain.

What works best is to practice these techniques until they're an ingrained habit rather than something you need to think too much about. Humans are creatures of habit. Consciously or unconsciously, we default to familiar ways of doing things. For example, when you brush your teeth, you're not thinking: *Okay, now for the right rear molar; okay, now the left. Up and down. Bottom to top.* Rather, you just do it because it has become habit at certain times of the day.

The same idea applies to meditation and other techniques. I can assure you that it gets easier as you go. The first time you practice meditating, it probably will not be as deep, effective, or familiar to you as it will when you've done it one hundred times. When your nervous system learns something new it reacts and responds differently than it does to the familiar. So when you sit down to meditate, embrace the positive—think about the steps you've taken in the right direction. As soon as you start focusing on how things aren't working, how they're out of control, how you don't know what's going to happen, you'll trigger a physiological state of anxiety—whether it's imagined or real.

Important message number one: *Don't get hung up on thinking that you don't have enough time to use these tools.* Even if you're just sneaking in a minute here and there to put them to work, or even if you can only afford or find time for one treatment with a practitioner every now and then. Of course two minutes are better than one and ten are better than five. But one is much, much better than none. So do a visualization exercise sitting in a parked car while Junior returns his overdue book to the library. Close your eyes and take yourself to a tropical beach. Inhale the scent of Coppertone. Feel the warm sand between your toes. My point? If you have just a few minutes, why not invest them in doing something that will make you feel good?

Important message number two: *Don't worry about getting it wrong.* Who ever gets anything right the first time? Not me, that's for sure. And that's the beauty of the four-week program. As you go along, you'll gain experience and you'll get better at every turn.

Kaizen, remember? Small steps.

METHODS OF ELICITING PEACE
AND RELAXATION

One of the prescriptions in my four-week program—in Part 3 of this book—is that you tap into some of the "pathways to peace" on a daily basis. So that you know what your options are—and so that you know how and why they work—here are the choices. You'll notice that I have broken them up into two sections: those you can do yourself and those for which you need a qualified practitioner.

Relaxation Exercises You Can Do Yourself

AROMATHERAPY

The sense of smell has a direct connection to the part of the brain that regulates mood—the limbic system. The power of aroma is evident in the way it can deeply affect emotions and conjure up memories. If you've ever strolled past someone wearing the same perfume your mother always wore, you'll know what I mean. In less than a nanosecond, images of Mom come flooding back. For many people the aroma of hot dogs recalls a certain baseball stadium, pine brings back summer camp, and the scent of freshly mowed grass has them dreaming of a golf course. There's more to aroma than memories, though.

Aromatherapy is based on the healing properties of plants from which highly concentrated aromatic oils are extracted. To give you an idea of *how* concentrated: it takes 220 pounds of lavender flowers to make about one pound of lavender essential oil. Some of the more commonly used oils are roman chamomile, geranium, lavender, leon, cedarwood, and bergamot. Each has a different chemical structure that affects how it smells and how it is absorbed and used by the body.

Essential oils can be used and enjoyed in one of two ways: you can inhale them or rub them into your skin. When inhaled, the vapors of the oils are carried via the bloodstream to the nervous system and to the parts of the brain that stimulate the release of neurotransmitters. When essential oils are massaged into the skin the results are the same. For a quick and easy way to unwind put a few drops on your pillow and rest your head there for a few minutes. Or put a few drops into a hot bath, lower yourself into the fragrant water, and, for a short while, shut off the world.

ESSENTIAL OIL BATHS were used in a study conducted at the University of Miami Miller School of Medicine.[3] A group of mothers gave their infants a bath with or without lavender-scented oil. The mothers in the lavender-bath-oil group were themselves more relaxed, and they smiled and touched their infants more often during the bath. Their infants looked at them for a greater percentage of the bath time, cried less, and spent more time in deep sleep afterward. As a bonus, the cortisol levels of this group of mothers and infants significantly decreased, confirming the data from many previous studies that showed the relaxing and sleep-inducing properties of lavender.

DAILY AFFIRMATIONS

Positive affirmations can be a powerful tool for reducing stress by increasing feelings of personal power. Talking to yourself in a positive manner can awaken your mind to possibilities for change. One type of affirmation combines autosuggestion and imagery. You articulate—silently or aloud—changes you'd like to see in your physical self, *as if they were happening in the moment*. You might say, for example, "I can feel my tension dissolving." "I feel calm." "Qi is quietly and freely flowing through my body." "My body feels warm, as if I'm snuggled under a down comforter."

Self-boosting affirmations work well, too. You can repeat them while falling asleep, or write them on a piece of paper and tape them to your bathroom mirror. Or, when you're taking your morning shower, write them on the glass door of your shower when it gets foggy. Then repeat them aloud as you're getting ready to take on the day. As part of the four week solution, you'll be asked to try some of these or create your own:

- I can handle whatever comes my way.
- Challenges bring opportunities.

- Little by little one walks far.
- Today has limitless possibilities.
- Today I will see things through a positive lens.
- When one door closes, another door opens.
- I have many friends and family who love and support me.
- I can accomplish anything.
- I am strong and the universe is my unlimited reservoir of energy.
- This too shall pass.
- My life is divinely synchronous.
- Obstacles present me with learning experiences and fade with insight.
- I am in charge of my life.
- I have many options.
- Every day in every way I'm getting better and better.
- I choose happiness.
- I open my heart and allow peace to fill my presence.

If you repeat an affirmation often enough, the thoughts eventually morph into self-fulfilling prophecies. As the images embedded in those suggestions become part of your subconscious, they will awaken the healing process. When you use affirmations, you're in a sense triggering endorphins, which means you're creating within yourself a sensation of happiness, safety, and well-being.

FOCUSED BREATHING

Breathing. You've been doing it since the day the doctor held you upside down in the delivery room and gently slapped your bottom. And my guess is, if you're reading this now, you've been doing it ever since. But there is breathing and there is *focused breathing*. We're here to talk about the latter.

Simple as it sounds, focused breathing—during which you think about your breath as you inhale and exhale—is a very effective stress-management technique. A slow, full breath triggers physical and cognitive changes that promote relaxation. Deep breathing helps release tension and anxiety and is a great energizer because the deeper the breath, the more your body is flooded with life-fueling oxygen. A full breath begins with the diaphragm pushing downward so that the stomach extends out. As your lungs fill with air, your chest expands. When you exhale, the reverse occurs—your chest settles first and then your stomach. Try this:

1. When anxiety strikes or you find yourself focusing on negative thoughts, immediately exhale through your mouth.
2. Now, open your lungs, and breathe in through your nose, drawing in a fresh, cleansing air to the count of four.
3. Exhale again slowly to the count of five.
4. Repeat four times.

MEDITATION

Meditation, one of the most commonly practiced mind-body interventions, is a mental exercise that induces relaxation and the physiological changes that accompany it. For people with SuperStress, the greatest benefit of meditation is the way it allows the mind to reverse the physiological effects of the stress response. Meditation done properly can slow your heart rate, breathing, and blood pressure. It ensures that you use oxygen more efficiently, and it diminishes the amount of cortisol produced by your adrenal glands and slows the rate at which your mind ages. Meditation has been scientifically shown to energize people who are sleep deprived, to improve concentration, and to strengthen the very structure of our brains as we age. As a SuperStress intervention, meditation can restore your body to a calm state, encourage self-repair, and prevent new damage due to the physical effects of stress.

Of the many approaches to meditation, the three most popular in the United States are mindfulness meditation, Transcendental Meditation, and focused meditation. Mindfulness meditation, which is rooted in the teachings of Buddhism, is based on the concept of awareness and total acceptance of the present. While meditating, you're directed to bring all your attention to the sensation of the flow of the breath in and out of the body. The goal is to focus attention on the present and the sensations you're feeling in that moment.

Transcendental Meditation, which originated in India, uses mantras (a word, sound, or phrase repeated silently) to prevent distracting thoughts from entering the mind. Popularized in the West by

Ayurvedic medicine's Maharishi Mahesh Yogi, Transcendental Meditation is a blissful relaxer. Meditators who engage in this practice are given a mantra by a teacher (or select their own) and repeat it while letting their minds drift naturally and effortlessly into a heightened state of awareness. Numerous studies of Transcendental Meditation have tested its effectiveness in countering stress. In one study[4] two groups were evaluated for hormonal changes in response to specific stressors before and after four months of either learning the Transcendental Meditation technique or generalized education on how to manage stress. The results showed significantly different results. In the group who practiced meditation cortisol levels decreased, but cortisol levels remained the same in the members of the group who studied conventional relaxation techniques. Overall, the results appear to support previous data suggesting that repeated practice of Transcendental Meditation reverses some of the physical effects of chronic stress.

Focused meditation is just as it sounds. You focus intently on a single object as a way of staying present in the moment.

How to Meditate

1. Find a quiet place and sit in a comfortable position. Progressively relax all the muscles in your body, and if it feels comfortable to you, close your eyes (unless you're doing focused meditation—see below).
2. Choose a word, phrase, prayer, or object that has special meaning to you or makes you feel peaceful—or just concentrate on your breath.
3. Breathe slowly and naturally. Inhale through your nose then hold the inhalation a few seconds. Exhale through your mouth, again pausing for a few seconds at the bottom of your exhale. Silently say your word, phrase, or prayer as you exhale. Repeat.
4. As you finish, continue to focus on your breathing as you sit quietly. Becoming aware of where you are, slowly open your eyes and get up. (If you have to keep track of the time, try using an alarm or timer set on the lowest volume, so you don't have to keep looking at your watch or clock.)

ALTERNATELY, YOU CAN TRY FOCUSED MEDITATION. Before you begin, select an object to direct your attention on—something small enough so that you really need to focus to see it. I use a statue of Buddha that's just one centimeter (about half an inch) high. Train your full concentration on the object for ten minutes. As thoughts come into your head, try to dismiss them and bring your attention back to your object of choice.

Practice for ten to twenty minutes per day, for at least three to four times a week.

Kirtan Kriya Meditation

Kirtan Kriya is an exercise that can boost your mental energy, creativity, and intuition. It employs four utterances that in Hindu tradition are associated with the stages of life.

> *Saa* is birth. Repeating the word calls to mind the most vibrant and vivid sensations that you have experienced: awakening to a view of a landscape covered in new-fallen snow; the opening bars of a beautiful symphony.
>
> *Taa* is life. Recall a loving experience, whether a deeply meaningful sexual experience or another profoundly intimate, tender moment, such as when your loved one reaches for your hand in the midst of a crowded room.
>
> *Naa* is death or completion. Envision a moment of great joy at accomplishing something you've worked very hard to finish, which you recognize as a great achievement.
>
> *Maa* is rebirth. Visualize a place of great beauty or great majesty, such as a centuries-old cathedral you have visited for the first time or a snow-capped mountain range as seen from an airplane.

With practice, these four sounds, chanted in order, will immediately bring to mind the feeling or image you've evoked for each. Chant *Saa Taa Naa Maa* while sitting cross-legged, with your back straight and your concentration focused. Imagine the sound flowing in through the top of your head and out the middle of your forehead, through the area known as the third eye. For two minutes, chant in your normal voice. For the next two minutes, chant in a whisper. Then for the next four minutes, chant silently. Then reverse the order, whispering for two minutes and then chanting out loud for two minutes, for a total of twelve minutes.

As you pronounce each syllable, perform the following finger exercises, which are a critical part of the meditation:

On *Saa,* touch the index fingers of each hand to your thumbs.
On *Taa,* touch your middle fingers to your thumbs.
On *Naa,* touch your ring fingers to your thumbs.
On *Maa,* touch your little fingers to your thumbs.

When you've completed the twelve-minute exercise, inhale deeply, stretch your hands above your head, and bring them down in a sweeping motion as you exhale. Kirtan Kriya is far easier than you might expect. With a little practice, you'll find it effortless and highly meaningful. Those wishing to learn more about this can see Dr. Dharma Singh Khalsa's website at www.drdharma.com.

PLAY TIME: IT'S NOT JUST FOR KIDS ANYMORE

We spend so much of our modern lives rushing from one place to another, always with an agenda, always believing that we've got to move on and get to the next appointment on our schedule. Do any of us ever really step back and reflect on the here and now?

It's important for everyone, but particularly for the SuperStressed individual, to have at least one activity you can pull out of your "toy box" and have fun with.

Play. Go on. You remember how to do it.

Playing provides a perfect way to express your creativity, to feel free in the moment, or just to blow off steam. When you are engrossed in an activity you enjoy, you can experience a state of being known as flow, in which your brain is in a near-meditative state. Proposed by positive psychologist Mihaly Csikszentmihalyi, the concept of flow has been widely studied. Its benefits include positive influences on body, mind, and soul.

Playing means stepping outside your daily routine and seeing things from a different perspective. You can do this in many ways. You can play with your kids or borrow their yo-yo for a half hour. Go to the park and swing on a swing and see how high you can go. Sit on the edge of a sandbox and remember what it was like not to worry about getting sand in your shoes.

There are additional ways to play—more serious ways—that will tackle your stress while simultaneously benefiting you and others. Volunteer at Habitat for Humanity and learn how to build a house. Read to a child. Read to yourself. Nothing takes your mind off stress like a good book, and you can go at the pace that seems pleasurable to you. Gardening is a great way to play; it recruits your senses and at the same time beautifies your surroundings and lets you connect with nature. Listening to music is another effective stress-busting hobby. Music provides inspiration as well as distraction. It can calm you down (or step you up), and it can keep you company at any time as you go about your day.

I'm playing right now as I list for you all these wonderful opportunities. And I would love to keep going. But the best part of playing is using your own imagination and dreaming. Why would I want to spoil your fun?

PETS CAN BE A SOURCE of comfort, solace, and joy to humans. They give us unconditional love, and they bring out our empathy, compassion, and nurturing skills. Pets can draw us out of ourselves and their presence increases mental stimulation by encouraging verbal and physical interaction. Many studies evaluating mood in relation to pet ownership have been encouraging, with results showing pet owners to have lower blood pressure, less heart disease, and to be less lonely. Some hospitals have added pet therapy—with highly trained socialized dogs, for instance—for their patients! For those who feel inclined and have the needed time, owning the right pet can be a truly rewarding experience.

PROGRESSIVE MUSCLE RELAXATION

This stress-relieving exercise cycles you through tensing and releasing moments and can help you identify where you hold stress in your body (for example, if you're one of the many people who sit hunched over a computer all day, you probably feel some tension across your shoulders). With this technique, you'll soon be able to identify exactly which body parts are most affected by the stress. At that point, you can concentrate on relieving the tension in those areas.

Even if you are active all day, this exercise is calming, introspective, and a good management technique for SuperStress. You might consider reading the following instructions into a tape recorder with a soft music background—voilà, you've just made your first self-help audiotape.

1. Start by raising your eyebrows as high as possible. Let the tension build and hold it for a moment.
2. Relax, and feel the tension flow out.
3. Squeeze your eyes shut as tight as you can and hold as the tension builds. Then relax your eyelids.
4. Clench your teeth together tightly and feel the tension building. Hold it for a few seconds and release.
5. Squeeze your whole face up hard, hold it, and then relax.
6. Turn your right hand into a tight fist and hold it, then release and feel the tension flow out through your fingers.
7. Do the same with your left hand.
8. Pull in your stomach muscles as tight as you can. Hold it while the tension builds and then relax.
9. If you're lying down or sitting in a chair, raise your right leg straight out in front of you, tensing your thigh and calf muscles and flexing your foot. Feel the tension build as you hold your leg up. Then, let your leg drift back down and relax.
10. Do the same thing with your left leg.
11. Tense your entire body and hold for several seconds, then release and sense the peaceful feeling you get from the relaxed state you have unlocked from this tensing exercise. Inhale and hold it for the count of four. Exhale, and as you do, blow out any remaining exhaustion in your body. Now open your eyes, and stretch your arms and legs for a few moments, enjoying the peace and comfort you feel.

TAI CHI

No doubt you've seen it before. Perhaps during a stroll through a park in the morning or through the doorway of a classroom at your local gym, you've witnessed a group of people performing a series of flowing movements in such slow motion that to watch them is to become instantly mesmerized. This is tai chi, a balance and flexibility technique that is sometimes referred to as focused inner peace through movement. In one sense, tai chi is a form of meditation. In another, it's low-impact yoga. The slow, gentle swaying movements, deep breathing, and mental focus of this exercise are designed to relieve tension, open up the joints, and allow chi, also known as qi, to move effortlessly throughout the body.

There's little gear required for tai chi. All you need are flat shoes, a four-by-four space, and a good teacher, instructional book, or video. (You can even skip the shoes!) Researchers exploring the benefits of this discipline have confirmed that tai chi can improve breathing, reduce stress, lower blood pressure, and correct balance. In one such study,[5] forty-eight male and forty-eight female tai chi students were randomly assigned to four treatment groups. For the purposes of the study, one group performed tai chi, and another engaged in a brisk walking exercise for the same amount of time as the tai chi group. The third group performed meditation, and the last group spent the time quietly reading. All participants were asked to perform mental challenges such as arithmetic (without pen and paper) and then they were shown a film that was intended to produce emotional disturbance. The results of the study showed that heart rate and blood pressure for those in the tai chi group were found to be better than for those in the last two groups and were similar to those who walked briskly. This tells us that tai chi is not only a meditative exercise but also one that has the same physical benefits of more strenuous exercises.

It's hard to describe in words the feelings you experience when practicing tai chi. I guess the best example is to liken it to my favorite sport, underwater diving. When you're diving, the minute you break the water, you find yourself in a totally different zone; a realm of sur-reality where you're quiet, yet moving; cocooned by the water, observing the blueness, the plants, and the fish as they glide silently by. Alone in the kingdom of calm, present in the moment. When you surface, you are renewed and you feel at peace, which is how you feel when you're in the zone of tai chi.

VISUALIZATION

One of the most common mental traps SuperStressed people fall into is forgetting that they have choices. In a sense we've become victims of our own decisions—to work late every night, to leave our PDA or BlackBerry on all the time, to overschedule ourselves, and to put sleep last on our "to do" list. Visualization exercises remind us that we have a choice as to how we look at things. When you are in a state of Super-Stress, you're often operating in the future or the past—agonizing over the botched pitch you made in the weekly editorial meeting or worried about the next deadline. Visualization brings you into the present because it requires your awareness of who you are and what you want to be. Through patterns of repetition, visualization allows you to create your own perception of reality.

To engage in visualization, you first must be in a relaxed state, which allows you direct access to your subconscious mind. Here are some steps to get you started.

- Find a quiet place and sit in a comfortable chair or lie down.
- Begin by focusing on your breath and breathing. Take several focused breaths as outlined on page 67 (this activates the vagus nerve, which is the major quieting nerve in the body).
- When you feel relaxed, begin by visualizing any scenario that will calm your mind and bring your awareness back to the present.

You can change your scenario as often as you like. I have a favorite one that I find myself repeating quite often.

1. I picture myself sitting serenely on the ground and leaning against an ancient tree.
2. I picture that the area where I sit is surrounded by wildflowers or small shrubs.
3. I imagine for a moment that I am connected to the tree from my tailbone to my skull along my spine.
4. I feel my head drawing sunlight down from the treetop, and I stretch my legs out straight, pressed into the earth, to draw nourishment from the roots of the tree. Connecting energetically to the earth literally grounds a person.
5. If any troubling thoughts, incidents, or encounters come to my mind, I visualize a flower in my hand. Then I place the incident or thought on its petals and give it away to the roots of the tree so that the negative energy can be released into the earth.

YOGA

If you've never practiced yoga, the word might conjure the image of someone sitting on the floor, legs crossed Indian style, hands in prayer position at heart level, sounding a long and generous "*ommmmmm*." Or maybe you think of a rubber-limbed maharishi standing on one leg, with the other gracefully wrapped around his neck. Both are indeed yoga poses, or asanas. But of course there's far more to yoga than assuming physical positions. Yoga is a blending of body, mind, and spirit—in fact, the word *yoga* comes from the Sanskrit word *yuj*, which means union.

No one really knows how old the practice of yoga is. Some say it may be as much as five thousand years old. It was originally developed as a discipline to help people reach spiritual enlightenment. The body movements and behaviors that make up this discipline—including conscious breathing, focusing attention, and maintaining a specific posture—are intended to suspend the stream of thoughts and relax the body and mind.

Hatha yoga, the type most commonly practiced in the United States and Europe, emphasizes postures (asanas) and breathing exercises (pranayama). Some of the major styles of hatha yoga include *Ananda, Anusara, Ashtanga, Bikram, Iyengar, Kripalu, Kundalini,* and *Viniyoga.*

People use yoga therapeutically for a variety of health conditions including anxiety disorders, stress, asthma, high blood pressure, and depression. They also partake of the discipline as part of a general health regimen to achieve physical fitness and to relax. Yoga is generally considered safe, but there are some situations in which the positions can pose a physical risk. Check with your doctor before starting a program, particularly if you have not done it before.

Methods for Which You Need a Therapist

ACUPUNCTURE

Acupuncture, one of the key components of traditional Chinese medicine, is among the oldest healing practices in the world. (Anything that's been around for 2,500 years deserves some kind of a medal, don't you think?) According to a 2002 National Institutes of Health (NIH) survey, an estimated 8.2 million American adults used acupuncture that year, up from 2.1 million the previous year.[6] A 400 percent rise is a story in itself!

Acupuncture is based on the traditional Chinese medicine premise that qi, the body's bioenergy system, travels through the body along energy channels called meridians, the way the veins carry blood around the body. Any interruption or blocked flow of qi leads to an imbalance in the forces of yin and yang, which ultimately disrupts well-being. The intention of acupuncture is to stimulate specific points on the body, primarily through the insertion of very fine metal needles, in order to clear any blocks in the flow of qi, thereby restoring balance and health.

While acupuncture has mystical origins, modern research shows that the practice makes biological sense. The effects of acupuncture likely come from the conduction of electromagnetic signals at a greater than normal rate. Those signals appear to stimulate the release of natural painkilling chemicals—endorphins—that automatically enhance feelings of wellness. Opinions vary a bit, but the consensus is that there are twelve main meridians and eight secondary meridians carrying qi, many of which flow through the major organs. A needle inserted in the wrist may affect your lungs because a meridian connects the two, encouraging the flow of qi. If you choose to include acupuncture as one of your relaxation techniques, make sure you see a well-recommended practitioner.

MASSAGE

You don't need a scientific study to tell you that massage therapy enhances relaxation and reduces stress. If you're one of the lucky people who enjoy a professional massage from time to time, you know what I mean. I've never known anyone who, just after a massage, jumped up raring to get back to work. On the contrary, most people are incredibly relaxed—it's all they can do not to fall asleep on the massage table.

There are many types of body massage, the most common of which include deep tissue, Esalen, and Swedish massage. All the techniques consist of a therapist pressing, rubbing, and moving muscles and other soft tissues of the body, primarily with their hands and fingers. The aim is to increase the flow of blood and oxygen to the treated area and, according to the principles of traditional Chinese medicine, to help unblock qi.

SuperStressed people respond positively to massage because the slow, rhythmic, and hypnotic strokes, often accompanied by soothing music, relax both the mind and body. That's because massage stimulates the release of mood-enhancing biochemicals, such as serotonin and endorphins. Massage can also boost mental and physical powers and improve quality of life for just about everyone. A recent study bears this out. Researchers from several institutions, including the Touch Research Institute at the University of Miami, have documented the positive effects of massage therapy on job performance and stress reduction.[6] The research, which evaluated twenty-six participants who had massage against twenty-four who did not, indicated that a basic fifteen-minute chair massage, provided twice weekly for five weeks, resulted in decreased job stress and significant increase in alertness and productivity.

REFLEXOLOGY AND AYURVEDIC FOOT MASSAGE

Reflexology is a specialized form of massage that focuses on the feet and hands. Practitioners learn the location of zones on the feet and hands, pressure sensors that are meant to communicate with the body's internal organs. Trained reflexologists map spots on the sole of the foot to particular corresponding organs, glands, and other body parts. Pressing on the right spot triggers a reflex reaction in the corresponding body part. For example, pressing on the ball of the foot can help problems in the heart or lungs.

Many of my patients find reflexology is an excellent means of reducing stress. Because the feet and hands help set the tension level for the rest of the body, they are a perfect place to intervene to interrupt stress signals and reset the body's equilibrium. In Indian reflexology, the foot is thought to have 107 principal junctions of ligaments, vessels, muscles, and bones called marmas. Reflexologists believe that massaging these marmas can eliminate toxins from the body. Whether that's true or not, it's still deeply relaxing. You can give yourself a foot massage with equally soothing results. When you rub your feet, you massage your whole body, balancing your emotions and improving blood and lymph circulation.

Guidelines for an Ayurvedic Foot Massage

1. Thoroughly wash your feet with soap and water, then wipe them dry.
2. Apply almond or sesame seed oil (not the cooking kind) infused with two or three drops of essential oil of lavender to one foot.
3. Start rubbing at the base of your little toe.
4. Continue at the base of the next toe over.
5. Apply slight pressure between your little toe and the next toe.
6. Now rub between that next toe and your middle toe.
7. Massage, stretch, and pull your middle toe in a circular motion.
8. Continue rubbing between and then massaging, stretching, and pulling your other two toes in a circular motion.
9. Apply gentle pressures to both sides of your heels below the ankles, then circle your ankles clockwise to boost energy and circulation.
10. Finally, massage your calf muscles to release tension.
11. Repeat on the second foot.

This Above All: *Don't Get Stressed Trying to Relax!*

You may know people who swear by yoga as the great be all, end all. And for them it may be—but remember that whatever relaxation technique you decide to try won't change your life overnight. They take practice, just as relaxation does, and that means weeks or months. Above all, *don't get stressed trying to relax*! If a particular exercise is not for you, try something else.

And don't forget to *breathe*.

CHAPTER FOUR

Foods That Heal

THERE IS NO DOUBT THAT STRESS IS a frequent visitor to the guest suites of the stomach and gastrointestinal (GI) tract. For the 1,402 people who reported stress-related physical symptoms in a recent major survey, the top three winners were fatigue (51 percent), headache (44 percent), and stomach-related problems including acid reflux and irritable bowel syndrome (34 percent).[1] But even though stress-related gastrointestinal difficulties took only the bronze medal, I have a feeling that many of the people who reported fatigue did so because they were poorly nourished or just plain hungry.

Are you convinced yet that you need to slow down? Of course. But we both know that's not always possible. In which case, the next best thing is to replenish the nutrients that are being lost to you.

And that in large measure is what the SuperStress Solution Diet is all about. Before we go farther, I want to make it clear that this isn't a stand-alone diet—none of these tools stands alone—but rather it's another bow in the quiver, a complement to the stress-reducing techniques we've read about in the last chapter and the ones that are still to come.

THE SUPERSTRESS SOLUTION DIET

The SuperStress Solution Diet is a meal plan that I designed to address every health- and food-related issue connected to SuperStress, including inflammation, nutritional depletion, and mood changes. For example, one of these issues is the continual release of cortisol into the body, triggered by the stress response. We're already well aware that stress hormones like cortisol rob the body of vitamins by commandeering them to support such classic stress responses as increasing the heart rate and the tensing of muscles. We also know that chronic stress-triggered cortisol in excess leads directly to belly fat—which, as we discussed in Chapter 1, is both unwanted physically and seriously dangerous to your health.

By reversing excess cortisol secretion and its undesirable effects, the SuperStress Solution Diet is not only going to help restructure your body, but will make you healthier in the balance, by attending to your nourishment needs. You'll retain all the vitamins you need to spirit you through your day. And here's the bonus: you'll probably shed a few pounds (or more) while you're gaining all the other benefits. Not a bad deal.

The SuperStress Solution Diet—which you will find in the appendix—includes foods that fall into three different categories: the Mediterranean Diet, Super Foods, and Mood Foods. To help you plan menus around these foods, I have organized two weeks of a regular diet as well as a weeklong detoxification plan, for those who choose to go that route. As you work through the four-week program in Part 3, you should be using these food plans at the same time.

THE FOUNDATION: THE MEDITERRANEAN DIET

The Mediterranean Diet is not a weight-loss plan like the fads you've read about or seen advertised on TV. I'm referring here to an eating style, one that is much like that of the countries surrounding the Mediterranean Sea. I chose the principles of the Mediterranean Diet as the foundations for the SSD because it's scientifically proven to be very healthy and because it addresses the kinds of body damage that occur with SuperStress. This type of diet reduces inflammation, replaces vitamins that are overutilized by bodies in a state of anxiety or stress, and provides enough fiber to support your gut and keep it healthy.

Part of the beauty of the Mediterranean Diet is that it is high in omega-3 fatty acids—essential nutrients found in fish, flaxseed, and nuts, which boost the immune system and reduce inflammation and depression, as well as stress.

Omega-3 fatty acids are also vital to the maximal function of cell membranes, specifically in the brain and the nervous system. More than 35 percent of the membrane tissue found in the brain comes from omega-3 fatty acids. Certain vision cells in the retina derive 60 percent of their fats from omega-3 fatty acids.

Omega-6 fatty acids play a role in the Mediterranean Diet, too. But unlike omega-3 fatty acids, omega-6 fatty acids come in healthy and unhealthy forms. Red meat contains the unhealthy form, and it is therefore highly inflammatory. Eggs, poultry, cereals, vegetables, and soybeans contain the healthy form, as do several oils you might not already have on your shelf but that you'll learn more about soon: borage oil, black currant seed oil, and evening primrose oil. These oils have anti-inflammatory properties.

The correct ratio of omega 3 and omega 6 in your diet has a calming effect and is particularly good for anyone who suffers from the symptoms of SuperStress. In recent decades, the typical American, through eating corn-fed livestock and genetically modified and processed foods, has come to consume twenty (or more!) times the amount of omega-6 as omega-3 fatty acids. Just as a measure of comparison, the ratio on which our ancestors thrived was closer to 1:1. Research now suggests that a 1:4 ratio of omega 3 to omega 6 may be best for defusing the stress circuit. This is the ratio we strive for in the SuperStress Solution Diet.

Mediterranean Diet Delectables

The Mediterranean Diet includes the following classifications of foods.

FRUITS AND VEGETABLES provide folic acid, B_6 and magnesium, which are required to boost the amino acids that improve mood. Seven servings a day are good; more are better. Variety is important, too. Different colored vegetables and fruits contain different vitamins, many of which add antioxidant support to overall health. When we consume them together it maximizes their goodness. So consume purple, red, orange, yellow, and green vegetables frequently, and mix them up. This rich cornucopia of phytochemicals boosts the immune system and protects against disease.

FATS. The focus of the Mediterranean Diet isn't to limit total fat consumption but to make wise choices about the types of fat you eat. Those choices should be predominantly in the monounsaturated fats (MUFAs) such as olive oil, which has a very specific anti-inflammatory quality, and polyunsaturated fats (PUFAs), which contain the beneficial linolenic acid (a type of omega-3 fatty acid). Olive oil should be the oil of choice. In addition to being a rich source of MUFAs, which keep HDL (healthy) cholesterol high and LDL (unhealthy) cholesterol low, new research reveals that extra-virgin oil—the oil that comes from the first pressing—can keep arteries clear of clots. When you buy olive oil, look for a brand that says "extra-virgin" on the label. The Mediterranean-type diet discourages (and the SuperStress Solution Diet prohibits) saturated fats and hydrogenated oils (trans-fatty acids), both of which contribute to increased inflammation and the formation of many chronic diseases such as heart disease, Alzheimer's, and type 2 diabetes. Extra-virgin and virgin olive oils are the most healthful because they are the least processed, so they contain the highest levels of the protective plant compounds that provide antioxidant effects. Oleic acid, which is a monounsaturated fat that is found in high concentration in olive oil, is more resistant to oxidation, and oxidation is how inflammation creates damaging effects on the body. Oleic acid has been shown to lower LDL and increase HDL. Compared to polyunsaturated oils like corn, safflower, and soy oils, olive oil can withstand heat; it and canola are the best cooking oils.

SMALL PORTIONS OF NUTS. Nuts may be high in fat (80 percent of their calories come from fat), but tree nuts—including walnuts, pecans, almonds, and hazelnuts—are low in saturated fat and have impressive cholesterol-lowering powers. Walnuts also contain omega-3 fatty acids. Nuts are high in calories, so they should not be eaten in large amounts—generally no more than a handful (¼ cup) or two a day. But nuts can be filling and stave off hunger pangs. According to a study published in the medical journal *Obesity*, Mediterranean citizens who ate nuts at least twice a week were 31 percent less likely to gain weight than those who ate them rarely or not at all.[2] For the best nutrition, avoid honey-roasted or heavily salted nuts. But peanut butter is acceptable, and even relished by most. (Yes! Peanut butter on a diet. What will they think of next?) However, those that really want to pack a punch should try cashew or almond butter, which contain a higher amount of omega-3 fatty acids.

RED WINE has two things going for it. It has an aspirin-like effect in that it reduces the blood's ability to clot, which is beneficial to the cardiovascular system. Red wine also contains an antioxidant known as resveratrol. Resveratrol is produced by plants in response to environmental stressors. It has been linked to reducing platelet aggregation, reducing inflammation, and blocking some cancer-promoting effects. Foods containing resveratrol include purple grape juice, mulberries, blueberries, bilberries and, in smaller amounts, peanuts. The Mediterranean Diet typically includes some red wine, consumed in moderation. This means no more than five ounces (a small glass) of wine daily for women (or men over age sixty-five), and no more than ten ounces (a larger glass) of wine daily for men under age sixty-five. Any more than this increases the risk of health problems. But wine has its downside, too. Excess alcohol can also increase the fat deposits in the heart, decrease immune function, and limit the ability of the liver to remove certain poisons from the body, including toxins produced during stress. If you don't drink, pure grape juice has proven to be just as effective at lowering total and LDL cholesterol.[3]

SMALL AMOUNTS OF RED MEAT. Red meat contains saturated fat. If you let a roast beef stand for more than an hour on a plate or cutting board, the liquid fat in the runoff juices congeals—much as it does in your arteries. Saturated fat augments inflammation by stimulating the arachidonic acid cytokine cascade. Substitute fish or chicken whenever you can and, when you do eat beef, mix it with whole grains and vegetables in stews.

FISH ON A REGULAR BASIS. Fish is a great source of omega-3 fatty acids. Omega-3 fatty acids lower triglycerides and LDL (the bad cholesterol) and may improve the health of your blood vessels. I recommend eating fish at least once or twice a week. Water-packed tuna, salmon, trout, mackerel, and herring—all oily fish—are the healthiest choices.

WHOLE GRAINS. Consumption of brown rice or barley increases tryptophan, which is an amino acid that promotes the production of serotonin, the hormone that gives you a sense of calm. When they are depressed, stressed, anxious, or SuperStressed, many people will load up on carbohydrates. Carbohydrate-rich meals trigger insulin production, which ultimately facilitates rising levels of tryptophan and serotonin in the brain. Eventually, the rise in serotonin shuts off the cravings for carbohydrates. Whole grains contain zinc, chromium, and magnesium as well as B_6, a vitamin that supports serotonin production.

Super Foods

Every indigenous culture includes foods of certain significance, either because these foods provide vital nutritive support or are integral to rituals that support and nourish our souls. The following is a list of the Super Foods in which I have indulged in my Micronesian travels and which I believe are manna for people with SuperStress, in part because they boost many of the key nutrients that have been drained as a result of being in the SuperStressed state. Just as important, these foods enhance our enjoyment of the sensation of eating and therefore relax us.

DARK CHOCOLATE. First on almost everyone's list of favorite foods is chocolate, which comes from the tropics and has a lot going for it in addition to its divine taste. For example, chocolate is plump full of flavanoids, a powerful class of antioxidants. Flavanoids have been shown to lower high blood pressure and reduce the risk of heart disease and strokes. Other compounds found in chocolate seem to lower the bad component of cholesterol (LDL) while leaving the good (HDL) component unchanged. Dark chocolate also contains several psychoactive chemicals that promote alertness and even euphoria. The latest scientific literature even shows it has some blood pressure–lowering properties.

To me, though, that's not what's so beautiful about chocolate. What I think is beautiful is its ability to enhance sensory recruitment in every way. It's so inexpensive to have a piece of chocolate and it's so pleasurable that if it's something you like I say: go for it. That's part of what living well is about. Once a day, treat yourself to a guilt-free one-third of a typical dark chocolate bar or one ounce of chocolate (roughly the size of the palm of a woman's hand). Doctor's orders!

COCONUT OIL has had a bad reputation in the West because it is 92 percent saturated fat, but its efficacy is currently being reevaluated. Coconut oil is a medium-chain triglyceride oil (MCT). MCTs have been used to improve the health of individuals with fat malabsorption problems. MCTs can be metabolized into usable forms of energy by the body almost as quickly as glucose. For people experiencing significant intestinal problems (bloating and cramps caused by high-fat foods), fatigue, and severe weight loss, I have suggested adding two teaspoons of coconut oil to a morning shake to boost calories and provide increased simple nutritive energy that does not create extra work for a damaged intestinal system. Additionally, the oil contains lauric acid, which is now recognized as an antiviral and antibacterial agent. Be aware, though, that one tablespoon of coconut oil contains 14 grams of fat and 115 calories.

COCONUT AND OTHER SPECIES OF PALMS are the foundation of the traditional Pacific Island lifestyle. The trunks are used for building and fuel; the fronds are woven into baskets and hats; and the outer husks with brown fiber (called coir) are twisted to make rope. The fine meshlike fiber at the base of each leaf is used as natural cheesecloth. Botanical medicines are pounded and placed in the fiber, which is then squeezed or rubbed over injuries, so that the plant sap will drip onto the skin. Because it ferments very quickly, the sap is also made into an alcoholic beverage called *tuba*. In Micronesia, coconut oil is used in cooking and when infused with essential oil of ylang ylang—a relaxing scent that I use in aromatherapy—as massage oil. Coconut oil is also the foundation of the first-birth ritual, among others. The first-birth ritual is a ceremony between families that socially welcomes the mother and newborn into the community. Over a period of days, the mother undergoes skin-softening botanical steaming and is rubbed with coconut oil and herbs by the women in the family.

CINNAMON. Islanders on the Micronesian island of Pohnpei brew a tea from ground local cinnamon bark (*Cinnamomum carolinense*) both as a household beverage and as a natural remedy for ailments ranging from backache to heavy menstruation. Other species (such as *Cinnamomun verum* and *Cinnamomum cassia*, the common spices found in our kitchens) have been shown to lower cholesterol and lower blood sugar, fight bacteria and a wide range of viruses, and promote the healing of wounds. Ongoing studies are examining cinnamon's anti-inflammatory, antibacterial, and even anti-cancer properties. Plus, it's delicious in everything from applesauce to stews!

TURMERIC. One of the principal spices in curries, bright yellow turmeric is used on the islands to treat skin ailments as well as in the first-birth ritual. In traditional Asian and Indian medicine, it is prescribed for everything from arthritis and amenorrhea to parasitic infections and ulcers. Modern-day research has shown that it has powerful anti-inflammatory and even cancer-fighting properties.

GREEN TEA. Tea—especially green tea—has long been known for its ability to revive, refresh, and relax at the same time. Tea also has an important component, L-theanine, which is a rare amino acid that stimulates alpha waves in the brain. Alpha waves are associated with relaxed, effortless alertness because they affect the balance of the mood-regulating neurotransmitters serotonin and dopamine. Tea is also a great source of flavanoids and antioxidants, which help to maintain cell health.

GINGER. Ginger has been used for thousands of years in Ayurvedic and Chinese medicine. Ginger contains anti-inflammatory, antibacterial, anti-ulcer, antiparasitic and antifungal properties. Ginger tea is soothing for stomachaches and is considered safe enough to be used to calm the nausea associated with pregnancy.

MOOD FOODS

The Food and Mood Project, a nutrition research group in the United Kingdom, has devised a classification of foodstuffs that it identifies as food *stressors* (foods that exacerbate stress from the inside) and food *supporters* (those that help people under stress). The lists were drawn on the basis of the personal experience among two hundred people who were enlisted to take part in this experiment.[4] Nearly 90 percent of those surveyed reported that when they changed their diet using these two categories as a guide, their mental health improved significantly. Participants reported that cutting down or avoiding food stressors like sugar (80 percent), caffeine (79 percent), and alcohol (55 percent) had the most impact on mental health. Additionally, improvements were reported when participants included more food supporters like water (80 percent), vegetables (78 percent), fruit (72 percent), and oil-rich fish (52 percent).

We've seen how certain foods help us to combat SuperStress. But it turns out that some foods can actually cause stress, too, because they alter our moods. Judith Wurtman, a professor at the Massachusetts Institute of Technology, has shown through years of research the ways in which certain foods alter mood by influencing the level of brain chemicals called neurotransmitters. Two neurotransmitters of interest to us—norepinephrine and serotonin—are influenced by certain foods and have opposing effects. Norepinephrine, which is in the adrenaline category, makes us more alert, while serotonin production has a calming effect.

Foods that increase norepinephrine are rich in protein and create a feeling of attentiveness, an increased ability to concentrate, and faster reaction times. These foods include tuna, turkey, and eggs. Eggs are especially beneficial because their yolks are rich in choline, an amino acid that enhances memory. (Choline deficiency is quite common, and some experts believe that a choline deficiency hastens the onset of Alzheimer's and other chronic memory loss syndromes. For those who cannot have egg yolks, wheat germ is another choline-rich food.) The foods that increase serotonin production are high in carbohydrates and include candy, cereal, bread, and pasta. The calming or anxiety-reducing effect of serotonin may be why we feel drowsy after polishing off a large bowl of spaghetti.

Endorphins are another group of chemicals that can affect both mood and appetite. Endorphins are the body's natural opiate-like chemicals that produce a positive mood, decrease sensitivity to pain, and reduce stress. A food substance related to endorphins is phenylethylamine, which is found in—guess what? Chocolate! Chocolate contains high levels of sugar and fat, phenylethylamine, and caffeine. The sugar in chocolate is associated with a release of serotonin, and the fat and phenylethylamine are associated with an endorphin release. This combination produces a calming, almost dreamy effect that has been called optimal brain happiness.

But before you rush out to buy a ten-pound bag of M&M's, you should know that any food-mood response is short-term. Eating a turkey sandwich at lunch may increase alertness and concentration, but generally only for two to three hours, just as having pasta with tomato sauce will produce a calming response for two to three hours. And then the party's over. Unless, of course, you choose to indulge again—which is not at all what I'm suggesting.

Bad Mood Foods

Much as I hate to admit it, too much chocolate can actually leave you sluggish after the sugar and caffeine jolts diminish. Likewise, an excess of potato chips drains the body and the brain, bringing on fatigue. And meals high in fat (read: fried chicken) raise stress hormone levels. Yet when we're in a bad or sad or mad mood, these are precisely the foods many of us reach for.

Two things in particular have few redeeming qualities: caffeine and sugar. While moderate amounts are acceptable, too much of either acts as a powerful stimulant to the body and hence can cause stress. Caffeine, which is found in coffee, tea, chocolate, and cola drinks, increases mental alertness and concentration and can improve performance, but taken in excess it has been associated with anxiety, cravings, depression, insomnia, and nervousness. As little as two cups of coffee, which amounts to approximately 300 mg of caffeine, has been reported to create a sense of anxiety. That's because caffeine promotes the release of adrenaline, thus increasing the level of stress. If you think about it, consuming too much caffeine might easily have the same effect as long-term stress.

Sugar doesn't have much going for it other than how absolutely wonderful it can taste. It has no essential nutrients. It has been linked to increasing inflammation—which, as we have already discussed, aggravates every symptom in a SuperStressed body—and it provides only a short-term boost of energy. Too much sugar too often can result in irritability, poor concentration, and depression. High sugar consumption puts a severe load on the pancreas and can lead to diabetes. It's best to try to avoid sugar, but if you find you cannot, then try to keep your blood sugar constant by not using sugar as a pick-me-up.

You can avoid the highs and lows of mood and energy associated with fluctuating blood sugar levels by choosing foods that are digested slowly. These foods have a low glycemic index and include whole-grain rye bread, oats, and rice.

Good Mood Foods

Certain vitamins, such as vitamin B_6, magnesium, folic acid (folate), and vitamin B_{12}, are essential for supporting the production of the feel-good brain chemical serotonin. Other mood-enhancing vitamins are vitamin C, which has been correlated with reducing the physiological stress effects of elevated cortisol, and zinc. Zinc is essential for those with SuperStress because it reverses some of the physiological stress effects of malabsorption, diarrhea, and glucose intolerance. Signs of zinc deficiency include anorexia, mental lethargy, irritability, low sperm count, generalized hair loss, rough and dry skin, slow wound healing, decreased thyroid function and a poor sense of smell. Many of the symptoms just mentioned are also common medical problems in stressed individuals.

Here are some other foods that stand out as mood elevators.

OATMEAL. Oatmeal may help if you find yourself feeling irritable and cranky. It is rich in soluble fiber, which helps to smooth out blood sugar levels by slowing the absorption of sugar into the blood. Oatmeal is also a great food to help you stick with your diet plan, because the soluble fiber in oatmeal forms a gel that slows the emptying of your stomach so you don't feel hungry quickly and it's high in our mood-soothing amino acid, tryptophan. Other foods high in soluble fiber are beans, peas, barley, citrus fruits, strawberries, and apples.

WALNUTS. Walnuts have long been thought of as a "brain food" because of their wrinkled, bi-lobed (brainlike) appearance. But now we know that walnuts are an excellent source of omega-3 essential fatty acids, a type of fat that's needed for brain cells and mood-lifting neurotransmitters to function properly and possibly to help some people with depression. Other foods rich in omega-3 fatty acids include salmon, sardines, flaxseed, and omega-3 fortified eggs.

TEA. Although caffeine has been shown to lead to a more positive mood and improved performance, there's a fine line between just enough and too much. Too much caffeine can make you dependent and nervous, irritable, and hypersensitive, or bring on headaches. Because brewed tea is lower in caffeine per cup than coffee, you can drink more tea than coffee before experiencing these effects. Tea also provides a little L-theanine, a calming amino acid.

SALMON. Sockeye salmon are an exceptionally rich source of vitamin D: a four-ounce serving of baked or broiled sockeye salmon provides 739 units, or 102 percent, of the daily requirements. In the past few years, research has suggested that vitamin D may increase the levels of serotonin, one of the key neurotransmitters influencing mood, and that it may help to relieve mood disorders.

LENTILS. A member of the legume family, lentils are an excellent source of folate, a B vitamin that appears to be essential for mood and proper nerve function in the brain. Low levels of folate have been associated with depression. In fact, a Harvard study showed that 15 to

38 percent of depressed adults are deficient in folate.[5] Although researchers don't yet fully understand the connection, folate deficiency appears to impair the metabolism of serotonin, dopamine, and noradrenaline, neurotransmitters important for mood. A cup of cooked lentils provides 90 percent of the recommended daily allowance of folic acid. A healthy bonus: lentils contain protein and fiber, which are filling and help to stabilize blood sugar.

CHAPTER FIVE

Rest and Motion

LIKE YIN AND YANG, REST and motion complement each other. A healthy mind and body require a certain amount of rest and a certain amount of motion. Too much of one without the other simply doesn't work. I've been saying this to my patients for years. "Get some rest," I suggest to the mother of twins who clearly doesn't carve out even a little time for herself. "You need more sleep," I say to the fourth-year surgical resident who complains that he's spent most of his residency "too tired to eat, too hungry to sleep." The mother of twins looks haggard. The surgical resident is operating—literally and figuratively—on far too little.

Just as often, I admonish patients to exercise more—or at least just move. "Get out of your car and *walk* a few blocks," I suggest to my female patient, a seventy-five-year-old suburbanite who never fails to be beautifully dressed but has put on several pounds a year for the past seven years. I also charge the young father who complains of lethargy to play ball with his sons as a way of energizing himself, blowing off steam, and keeping himself fit.

Rest, and its extension: sleep. Motion, and its extension: exercise. Both are essential not only for the SuperStressed, but for everyone. This chapter will help you understand why you need both and how to fit more of each into your busy days (and nights).

REST AND SLEEP

REST: RESTORING THE BODY

Rest is the conscious form of restoration. When you're resting, even though you're awake, your body is restoring itself. Think of rest as *the true state of awake stillness.* Think of the meditative exercises you read about in Chapter 3. Your body is letting go when it's at rest.

Of all the suggestions I make to my SuperStressed patients, the one that is the hardest for them to hear is this: Several times during your day, stop what you're doing, get up from your computer, turn off your cell phone, and rest for five or ten minutes. By the way they look at me, you would think I was suggesting they stop breathing. Why? Because *rest* is a word that SuperStressed people do not like. Though the questionnaire has perhaps helped you start to see things differently, think about it: wouldn't you say you don't *need* rest? Don't you think you're doing just fine?—even though you're constantly on the go, always behind, always in catch-up mode. And if by some stroke of luck you do catch up, don't you often just take on more, raising the bar higher and higher until it's virtually impossible to scale it? Unless you sacrifice something. Which, of course, you do. And what is the easiest sacrifice for a SuperStressed person to make? The one that buys us the most time?

Sleep.

But let's not cross the bridge to slumber just yet. Let's rest for a moment on the subject of rest. Nothing can survive without rest. You might think that lying in a hammock or reading a book is the definition of rest, but for me it's sailing, golf, or rock climbing. So who's right? We both are. That's because mental rest can be achieved through doing something you enjoy, something that lets your mind wander away from the everyday, mundane things on our plates.

Physically, rest gives our bodies time to repair cellular damage and absorb nutrients. But rest is also essential for our brains. If you've found yourself losing focus even when you're trying hard to pay attention, you know that the brain in its waking state needs time to drift, to daydream, and to wander. Our brains check out sometimes without our awareness— they take a little nap, and then we "wake up" and become present again. Smart fellow, that brain. It knows when it needs a rest, even if we don't.

Ernest Rossi, a specialist in medical hypnosis, explains this more scientifically when he describes a phenomenon known as *ultradian rhythm*. This is a natural cycle of repeated switching of brain hemispheric dominance, from left brain to right brain and back again. This switching occurs over a period of ninety minutes, during both waking hours and sleep. The left hemisphere is generally ascribed to logical thinking and the right is more adept at dreaming. The switchover itself, from one side to the other, takes around twenty minutes. Those twenty minutes are the body and mind's natural time for recuperation and may leave you feeling just the slightest bit drowsy. . . . Some people try to buck themselves up by having a cup of coffee or a candy bar. Rossi suggests that taking a small ten-minute break can mediate the stress of struggling to surmount this down time. You can get through it without a break—who has time for a break every ninety minutes?—but that's because the switch is going to happen again within a reasonable amount of time.

If you find yourself regularly struggling during the day to stay focused and to shake off drowsiness, consider taking a power nap, a ten-minute snooze at your desk or on a sofa—just a short period in which to fully give in to your sleepiness. A lot of people swear by them, and we are now learning that power naps may have tangible health benefits as well because you are reenergizing yourself in a natural way rather than requiring artificial stimulants such as several cups of coffee to keep you going. In lieu of a power nap, try some of the one-minute and five-minute relaxation exercises in Chapter 3.

SLEEP: RESTORING THE MIND

If rest is the conscious form of restoration, sleep is the unconscious form. In sleep, the mind is restoring itself by letting go of rational thought. Though the sleeping person is not aware of it, studies show that sleep is an essential part of the process of enhancing your learning and memory. Various sleep stages are involved in the consolidation of separate types of memories, and being sleep deprived reduces a person's ability to learn. All most of us know is that when we skimp on sleep, we don't function as well. And you can cover that up only so long.

From the safe haven of your apartment, or even from the bedroom, you might think: *Who will know if I don't sleep tonight?* If you live alone, no problem: no one will know. But if you live with someone or you're married, like my patient Suzanne, it's a lot harder. Suzanne was on the fast track to make partner at her law firm. Her work was piling up. Even after she brought work home to do when the kids were asleep, the pile kept getting bigger and her stress increased. Her husband, Jack, was growing impatient. She knew he wanted some of her time, too, so when Jack suggested they retire for the evening, Suzanne dutifully followed him up to bed. But when Jack was asleep, she padded downstairs and into the den to do just "one more hour" of work. That hour turned into four, and although she returned to the bedroom, she was never quite able to fall back into a healthy sleep. After several nights of this, she was so sleep deprived that she nodded off in her office. And on the bus. And at an opera she'd been looking forward to for months. She drank three cups of coffee to stay awake through the law firm's annual meeting, but she was clearly lackluster and unable to participate on an intelligent level. Not exactly partner material.

Nature's Sleep Cycles

Sleep has much to do with our biological rhythms, sometimes called *circadian rhythms*—a roughly twenty-four-hour cycle of the biochemical, physiological, or behavioral processes. Patterns in nature have developed by trial and error over millennia, and today's scientific tools are confirming their validity in relation to human sleep. We now know that the moon affects the movement of water and nutrients within different parts of plants and that there are direct correlations between plant growth and lunar phases. In addition to the lunar cycle, plants have internal rhythms that let them tell time and judge the optimal periods for flowering and germination, as well as when to expect bad weather.

Animals have similar cycles—and so do human beings. For example, our cortisol levels rise in the morning and peak at 9:00 A.M., which is why heart attacks are 30 to 40 percent more likely to occur between 6:00 in the morning and noon. Our blood pressure follows the same pattern, reaching its highest level in the morning and falling at night, when we get ready to go to sleep. But today, when so many of us are literally stewing in stress hormones, our cortisol levels are higher at all times of the day.

Some Insomnia-Fighting Strategies

Few situations are more frustrating than lying in bed wondering when you're going to fall asleep. But if you're one of the 20 million Americans who suffer from insomnia, you probably know by now that the direct route to a good night's sleep is to relax before bed. Toward that end, here are a few foolproof ways to ease the stress you have accumulated throughout the day and start to relax so that you might drift easily into a restorative sleep.

Tune out the day. You've likely spent all day working your brain, so let it rest before turning in for the night. Try some activities that involve low mental effort, such as stretching or listening to calm music.

Don't bring work home, but if you must, don't bring it into your bedroom, and if you *must* bring it into your bedroom, do not bring it into your bed. Working in bed sparks an accumulation of the stress hormone cortisol, which in turn makes falling asleep difficult.

Make sleep a priority. Staying out late on more than the rare occasion can stress the body by interrupting the restoration it requires. Think about yourself and your sleep when making evening plans.

Stay cool. When your body temperature is elevated, it's harder to stay asleep. Falling asleep is easier when your body temperature is at its lowest. The redistribution of heat from your core to your arms and legs induces relaxation and rapidly lowers the heart rate, prepping the body for sleep.

Relax to the beat. I've been intrigued by recent research on binaural beats, a therapy that has been shown to reduce anxiety and promote sleep. Binaural beats are tones heard through earphones. Each earphone emits a tone that is slightly different from the other with the result of two slightly different wavelengths reaching the brain. The change is imperceptible to the ear but the effect of these sounds is to change and entrain brain waves to facilitate relaxation and other health benefits. One study suggests the benefits of regular listening to binaural beats include reduced stress and anxiety, and increased focus, concentration, motivation, confidence, and depth in meditation.[1] I used a personalized version of this technique when treating Sara, a thirty-seven-year-old city planner from a large suburb of New York who held a senior position in city government. Sara had come to see me after three doctors were unable to remedy her many physical ailments.

Sara's Story

At some point, Sara had stopped deriving pleasure from her achievements, and on the eve of being reappointed to a new term by the mayor, she was having second thoughts about accepting the position.

It turned out that several years before, soon after launching a computerized system that kept tabs on all of the city's new construction and the construction companies, Sara had developed a serious case of eczema on her arms, chest, and face. For a year, she'd been on steroid creams to suppress the itch and on sleeping pills to help her fall asleep and stay asleep. Though she and her doctor recognized that the rash was stress-related, Sara couldn't soothe her anxiety. When her program began to get national attention, she developed severe pelvic pain, which was diagnosed as endometriosis. She had two surgeries to remove the encroaching tissue, but it kept advancing.

She came to my office believing that any high-profile success she achieved would exact a heavy toll on her health. She was also worried about her growing dependence on sleeping pills. As usual, I began by reviewing her options, including counseling. "You're not the first to suggest that," she said, but dismissed the idea as too time-consuming and also a political liability. "Can't we just do something here? Now? Between us?" she asked. "I'm willing to try just about anything."

I agreed. And I started by giving Sara a biofeedback tool called Biodots to monitor her stress levels for a week. The Biodot is a tool I often use as a barometer for reading stress levels. It is a small plastic dot the size of a hole left by a hole punch. The color of the Biodot can change when it's on your skin. I usually put it on the back of my hand. The colors change to reflect the temperatures that you generate in your skin, relative to diminishing blood flow through your blood vessels. When Sara was relaxed, the Biodot on her hand would be blue, and under severe stress, it would turn black. At our next appointment, she reported that the color never varied—the Biodot was always black. "Which tells us you were 'on' the whole week," I said. "Do you think you relax?"

"Of course I do."

"What do you do to relax?" I asked.

Sara said that after dinner (and sometimes during it) she watched TV, and at bedtime, she went upstairs and, after taking a sedative, usually fell asleep in her bed with the TV still on. That was a problem in itself because the screen light and noise were probably stoking her anxiety. We talked some more and drew up a plan.

"Okay," I said. "Here's what you need to do for the next three weeks." I told her to turn off the television at least an hour before bed and to make sure that there was no ambient light in her room at all, not even a night light. Then I changed her evening routine. After dinner, instead of turning on the TV, she was to take a long bath with lavender essential oil and drink a calming tea. Thirty minutes before bed, she would take 1 mg of melatonin. I suggested that we create a script for a tape of affirmations, which she would read over a background of her favorite music while doing a progressive relaxation exercise. The script we created, which was repeated four times on the tape, reflected Sara's own vision of serenity:

- I am calm and relaxed.
- I feel quiet.
- My whole body feels soft, relaxed, heavy, and comfortable.
- My mind is quiet.
- I withdraw my thoughts from my surroundings, and I feel serene and still.
- My thoughts are turned inward, and I am at ease.
- Deep within myself, I am relaxed, comfortable, and still.
- I feel a deep, inner quiet.

We created the tape together, but Sara resisted the idea of using it. "I don't know, Dr. Lee," she said. "First of all, I'm not sure I can sit still long enough to listen to this four times, and second, well, does this stuff really work?"

I urged her to try it, explaining that she wasn't just trying to sleep, but also learning to soothe her nervous system. The Biodot would show whether she was making progress.

Within a week, Sara called, as planned, and reported that the routine was "actually making a difference!" For several nights in a row, her Biodot had turned blue, and she awoke feeling refreshed. Now that she'd begun to access serenity and knew how it felt, I prescribed some brief relaxation sequences she could do during the day to keep her anxiety at bay. The combination of daily relaxation interludes and the nighttime routine paid off, and soon she was off the heavy-duty sleeping medications and on the road to deeper healing. (She kept her job, by the way.) She now tells me that her colleagues are hooked on Biodots.

There's a lot you can do to regain control over your sleep. Minor lifestyle and environment changes—such as preparing for sleep, following a sleep schedule, and making your bedroom conducive to sleep—can have a major impact. The following suggestions—both strategies and supplements—for healthy sleep have been endorsed and approved by my patients. Sweet dreams.

Chronic sleep disturbances include:

- Snoring
- Narcolepsy
- Restless leg (or arm) syndrome
- Chronic nightmares
- Periodic halt to breathing during sleep (sleep apnea)

If you experience any of these conditions regularly, especially if it has been troubling you for months, it's important to see a doctor prior to implementing the following sleep strategies just to make sure that your condition is not a symptom of some other illness such as depression, heart disease, or diabetes.

DR. LEE'S PRESCRIPTION FOR HEALTHY SLEEP

Improving Sleep Ambience

Let's start simple. Ambience refers to your surroundings as well as your activities prior to going to bed. Here are some ways to improve your sleep environment:

- Don't drink caffeine after dinner.
- Don't exercise within two hours prior to going to bed.
- Have as comfortable a mattress and pillow as possible.
- Use your bedroom only for sex or sleeping.
- Keep the room as dark as possible and if necessary, use a sleep mask. Ambient light disturbs sleep.
- Keep the sleep area as quiet as possible.

Sleep Rituals

If you repeat a thought or an action often enough, it soon becomes second nature. This works with falling asleep as well. Try to keep to these rules every night for four weeks.

- Keep on or as close to a regular sleeping and waking schedule as you can, even on weekends when possible.
- Make bedtime a relaxing, mind-clearing nightly ritual.
- Read a book (not anything related to work, though), listen to music.
- Perform a five-to-ten-minute relaxation exercise (see Chapter 3).
- Take a leisurely bath with essential oils such as
  - Lavender
  - Marjoram
  - Roman chamomile
  - Hops
  - Valerian
  - Vetiver
  - Clary sage
- Add two drops of one of the above oils to one teaspoon of vegetable oil to massage on your feet before bed.
- *Do not watch television in bed, and particularly do not watch TV news.*

Sleep Aids

These items are fairly easy to obtain but are so simple they are worth mentioning:

- White-noise machines are useful for drowning out periodic sounds such as neighbors' conversations and television sets, or outside traffic.
- Earplugs
- Sleep mask
- Warm socks. It's healthy and easier to sleep in a cool room, but at the same time, you may find your feet get cold. Warm feet tend to keep the whole body warm on chilly nights and so socks are the perfect answer.

Sleep Supplements

The following nonprescription supplements have been scientifically shown to be helpful in treating insomnia. Unless otherwise indicated, they are all available in pill or capsule form and can be purchased in most health food stores and pharmacies.

Melatonin

There are two kinds of melatonin on the market: sustained release and immediate release. Sustained-release melatonin is considered best for improving sleep maintenance. Immediate release is best for improving sleep *latency*—that is, reducing the time it takes to fall asleep. You should never take melatonin if you're going to need to drive or operate heavy machinery within four to five hours afterward (which you shouldn't be doing anyway—this is sleep time!), and you need to be aware that in addition to causing drowsiness (which is what you're aiming for), melatonin can also cause headaches and dizziness. For the SuperStressed, immediate release is the place to start.

DOSE: Take .5 mg to 5 mg in capsule or tablet form. Higher doses seem to produce a hypnotic effect. Expect to take this for two or three days before it begins to help with your insomnia.

ADVERSE EFFECTS: May cause excessive drowsiness.

If melatonin helps you fall asleep but you find you need additional sleep support to stay asleep, add one of the following herbs.

Valerian *(Valeriana officinalis)*

This herb has long been used as a remedy for insomnia. How it works in the body is not well understood but some studies suggest that it may affect levels of the calming neurotransmitter GABA. Clinical evidence shows that it reduces the time it takes to fall asleep and improves sleep quality.

DOSE: Take 400 to 900 mg in capsule form. Valerian works best when it is taken thirty minutes before bedtime. Expect results after several weeks of steadily taking valerian. Valerian can be used in combination with hops, skullcap, poppy, and lemon balm.

ADVERSE EFFECTS: Sometimes people report headache, stomach discomfort, and/or morning drowsiness.

If used in combination with sedative medications, valerian may increase drowsiness. It also has been known to occasionally cause vivid dreams.

Hops *(Humulus lupulus)*

Hops is used as a flavoring for food and also for beer. The flower is the part responsible for creating a calming effect.

DOSE: Take 41 mg (capsule or drops) prior to bed.

ADVERSE EFFECTS: Too much of this herb can cause sluggishness.

Kava *(Piper methysticum)*

This is more of a muscle relaxant than a sedating herb, but many of my patients feel it works well for them in concert with melatonin.

DOSE: Take 100 to 120 mg (70 mg kara-lactones) thirty minutes before bed. This preparation comes in capsule form and the active ingredients, known as kavalactones, should be included on the label.

RISK: Some people have had liver irritation and inflammation from this herb, so if you plan to use it regularly, make sure your doctor knows.

ADVERSE EFFECTS: May cause stomach upset. (Note: Avoid if taking other sedative medications.)

Lemon Balm *(Melissa officinalis)*

DOSE: Take 80 mg capsule before bed.

ADVERSE EFFECTS: Can cause extreme drowsiness if used in combination with other sedatives.

Skullcap *(Scutellaria lateriflora)*

DOSE: Take 1 to 2 mg in capsule form before bed or as a tea. Tea should be made with hot water and 1 to 2 ml tincture of skullcap. Take either capsule or tea thirty minutes before bed.

ADVERSE EFFECTS: None known at lower doses.

Passion Flower *(Passiflora incarnata)*

DOSE: Take as .25 to 2 g in capsule form or .5 to 1 ml of liquid extract in tea.

ADVERSE EFFECTS: Can cause dizziness.

California Poppy *(Eschscholzia californica)*

DOSE: This comes in the form of loose tea. Steep 1 tablespoon in ½ cup of water.

ADVERSE EFFECTS: Can cause morning sluggishness.

German Chamomile *(Matricaria recutita)*

DOSE: Take 10 drops liquid extract in a cup of warm water before bed.

ADVERSE EFFECTS: If you're allergic to flowers in the daisy

family, you may want to consult with your health care practitioner to see if this is safe to take.

Roman Chamomile *(Chamaemelum nobile)*

DOSE: Take 1 to 4 g of flower heads in a tea or 1 tablespoon in ½ cup water before bed.

ADVERSE EFFECTS: None known at lower doses.

L-theanine

DOSE: Take 100 mg capsule at bedtime.

ADVERSE EFFECTS: Excessive sleepiness if combined with other sedatives.

Saint John's Wort

For mild depression and depression-related insomnia.

DOSE: Take 300 mg capsule three times a day.

ADVERSE EFFECTS: Can cause an allergic rash if you are overly exposed to the sun. (Note: Avoid if taking antidepressants)

MOTION AND EXERCISE

Movement has always been a natural part of life and it has contributed evolutionarily to our survival. Our ancestors hunted and gathered, and later raised livestock and plowed fields. If they needed anything, they left the dwellings that they had built and went out to procure it. When the weather turned cold, they took off for the tundra in search of wood to burn. And how did they get to these far-off places? They walked, of course. Without an iPod, without Nikes. Without even a Reebok triple-nylon sweat suit. Can you imagine? All that our ancestors had were strong calf muscles, sharp vision, and a brain. They ventured forth every single day, because they had to. And that's because there was no refrigeration on the savannas and plains, so no matter how great one day's catch, by the next day it was not fit to eat. But let's say one of the pack decided *not* to go out. Let's say he decided to take a day off, maybe two. Okay, so he'd have to eat leftovers. But then the food supply would diminish. In short order, his brain would sense a famine coming, and would send a directive to his body to slow down and start conserving energy for the future. But here's what happens inside our stay-at-home's body as a result of slowing down: his metabolism drops, his energy flags, his muscles begin to melt, and his body starts to store fat, rather than burn it.

Is that what you want?

Move It!

Movement and exercise still work the same wonders they did for our ancestors, but we know so much more today about the benefits. Let's just take walking, for example. A fifteen-minute walk increases your blood circulation, which delivers oxygen and glucose to your brain, thereby clearing the head, so you're going to think well. Regular walking can improve your brain's "executive function," the ability to concentrate and act appropriately, and your working memory—even if you don't start exercising until your seventies. Walking is good for your blood vessels, your immune system, and your mood.

A study from Brigham and Women's Hospital in Boston found that women who exercised just two hours a week (or seventeen minutes daily) reduced their risk of heart disease and stroke by 27 percent.[2] And, adds Barry Franklin, Ph.D., director of cardiac rehabilitation and exercise laboratories at Beaumont Hospital in Royal Oak, Michigan, "You don't even have to do it all at once. No fewer than ten studies since 1995 show that breaking up physical activity into small segments of about ten minutes is just as effective."[3]

EXERCISE AND SUPERSTRESS: WHAT HAS ONE GOT TO DO WITH THE OTHER?

Exercise is an incredibly effective stress reliever. Virtually any form of exercise can decrease the production of stress hormones and counteract your body's natural stress response. Here's why. During exercise, the body naturally produces and releases the opiate-like chemicals called endorphins, which are nature-made to reduce the pain that comes with a hard workout. When produced in moderate levels, endorphins make you feel good—think of the "runner's high." But endorphins are not the only chemicals produced during a good workout. Neurotransmitters—mood elevators like dopamine, norepinephrine, and serotonin—are also produced. Low levels of those neurotransmitters can result in anxiety and depression. Exercise helps to keep the levels high enough to combat those feelings.

Exercise helps to reduce cortisol and other stress hormones. As you know, these hormones can harm the body if left in the bloodstream too long, and can cause a narrowing of the arteries, which can lead to a heart condition. Exercise breaks down these harmful hormones so that they can then be easily passed out of the body. Exercise also helps by increasing blood vessels' resilience, so that any harmful compounds that remain are less damaging.

SuperStressed people often have muscle tension in their neck, shoulders, or back. Certain exercises strengthen those muscles and increase their supply of fresh oxygen, making tension less likely after a workout.

Exercise can also serve as an outlet for frustration. When life's everyday aggravations build up, both high- and low-energy forms of exercise can release these negative emotions. Focusing on an exercise takes your mind away from the problem that is causing you stress and turns it toward doing something good for yourself. The effect of this is *homeostasis*. Remember we spoke of balance in Chapter 1? By this same principle, your body is brought back to a state of equilibrium, or its natural state, which is free of worries and stress.

Are you convinced? I hope so. Because I can't tell you how many of my patients are full of excuses: "I'm just too busy to exercise. No way can I spare an hour to go to the gym." And it's not just my *patients*.

"I *Hate* the Gym!"

I have a friend who hates the gym. Pure and simple. If an Oscar or a Pulitzer or some such award were given for the most original reasons not to go to the gym, Allison would win it. The dog ate her sneakers. Her car was repossessed. She has had dentist appointments, blind dates, even an overdue book report. Allison loves to eat, shop, talk, sing, and play Scrabble. But exercise? She just doesn't like it. And she doesn't much like me, either, when I try to tell her that she needs to do it anyway. Of course, I'm careful to explain that exercise is not something that she can only do in a gym. A gym is the twenty-first century's format for exercise—along with wearing the right outfits and working out with the right trainer. And yes, belonging to the *right* gym, for heaven's sake. But the reality is that exercise can be done anywhere as long as it involves the body in motion. It's walking in the park, climbing a tree, dancing, swimming, or playing golf.

You don't have to spend an hour on the treadmill to reap the benefits of exercise. Studies show that small, incremental bursts, such as three short, brisk walks—in the morning, at lunchtime, and in the evening—benefit you nearly as much as thirty straight minutes of sweating and slogging. Who can't find a few ten-minute patches in their day?

Come on. You know you can!

If you recall, a critical step in Chapter 3, "The Pathways to Peace," is making time for your own self-care—and not necessarily the back-to-back hours that so many of us who live in the twenty-first century believe we can't spare, but smaller pockets of time dedicated to improving your well-being. If you must, think of exercise as a job and show up for work every day. If you consistently—or even often—called your boss and asked for a day off, how long do you think you would last in that job? Commit to yourself. Five-minute pockets, six times a day. Ten minutes, four times. Do it like brushing your teeth. Do it automatically.

Just do it.

Below you'll find a series of exercises that both the scientific literature and my patients will tell you will counteract your SuperStress, build strength and self-esteem, and are enjoyable. Among these are a no-gym workout program and an offering of mix-and-match exercise prescriptions—ways to increase your movement a few times during your busiest days, as well as twenty-minute programs for the days when you have a lunch hour.

Before you begin, you should consult with your health care provider, especially if you have a history of heart disease or other risk factors. Remember to build up your fitness level gradually. It's safer, and if you begin your program slowly, you are more likely to stick with it. Finally, don't think of exercise as optional. Think of it, as I said earlier, as as an opportunity to affirm your worth and show up every day.

Dr. Lee's Prescription for SuperStress-Busting Exercises

By now we're all pretty well schooled in the many ways exercise benefits the body. Exercise provides immeasurable benefits for the mind, too, particularly the minds of SuperStressed individuals. Physical exercise decreases the production of stress hormones by counteracting your body's natural stress response. As you begin to shed your daily tensions through movement and physical activity, you may find that the resulting energy and optimism it brings can help you remain calm and clear.

I know, I know. No one loves to stop what he or she is doing and hit the trail. So, I'm going to make this as painless and as easy as possible—mostly because I want you to partake. That's how important I think exercise is. My suggestions come in two categories, both of which have the same intention: to take the *stress* out of *SuperStress* and leave you feeling, well, *super*.

TIMED WORKOUTS (which include walking) are designed to fit into your busy day. Even if you have only several small pockets of free time, you can wedge mini-workouts into them.

VENUE CHOICE EXERCISES. I have proposed a series of exercises that can be done both inside your home or outside (or both).

So you won't get bored undertake something from each category on alternating days for variety—which is proven to help you stick to your exercise commitment. Take along an iPod or a friend.

You'll also note at the end of this chapter a series of stretches which I believe are helpful for both relaxation and flexibility. Stretching is an excellent antidote to SuperStress. Try to stretch before you begin exercising and, if time permits, again afterward. Even if you're not exercising but just feel "tight," you can count on these stretches to help you relax. Try it!

Exercise Tips

- The best way to tackle exercise is to start slowly and build up until you reach a level of fitness you're comfortable with.
- Don't overdo it at the beginning. Work hard enough so that you feel as if you're doing something fun but still getting a health benefit.
- Step up the pace a little each week, and soon you will be in an exercise groove.
- Most important, check with your doctor before you begin any exercise program.

TIMED WORKOUTS

Just because you can't commit to a daily uninterrupted half hour or more of exercise doesn't mean that you can't get any benefit. When it comes to stress management, every morsel of exercise counts. Really. Any activity (even stretching) that gets your heart pumping makes your endorphins flow and relieves stress. Studies have shown that if you perform only five minutes of reasonably intense exercise in the morning, you can potentially burn up to twice as many calories as you normally would during the day![3]

What all this means is that "I don't have time!" is no excuse anymore. Five minutes a whack—that's all it takes. Toward that end, here is a series of exercises that you can do if you have five minutes or more. Some are aerobic, some are stretching, and some improve your balance. All are designed to relieve your stress and enhance your mood.

Note: All quoted rates of calorie burning will depend on your weight and gender.

FIVE FIFTEEN-MINUTE WORKOUTS

In and Around the Home

Walk! Walking is wonderful. It gets you outdoors (though you can certainly walk around an indoor track or a mall—many people do!), burns calories, strengthens your legs and calves, improves your circulation, keeps your joints lubricated, and builds stamina. Oh, and it's a lightning-fast way to reduce stress! Finally, it's free, and can be done anywhere. All you need is some motivation and a good pair of walking shoes.

The average American walks from 4,000 to 5,000 steps per day (depending on which study you read) without much thinking about it. That's around two miles in the form of walking around your office, walking to the mailbox, walking your dog, and walking around your house. To combat SuperStress, I am not asking you to increase this amount by much: my recommendation is to work up to around 7,500 steps a day to show maximum benefit. (And 7,500 steps a day will knock off the pounds, too, in case you're interested.)

Using a pedometer will tell you how many steps you're taking. They are available in most sporting goods stores, come in all shapes and sizes, and are not terribly expensive, and they work. Just strap one on to your belt in the morning and go about your day. By evening, you'll know how many steps you've taken. Because some pedometers can be more finicky than others, I suggest that you record your steps daily for a week and then average them out. Studies show that being conscious of the number of steps taken is enough for some people to get moving and add to their normal amount of steps. Remember, if walking does a good job of reducing stress—which we know it does— then walking more does a better job. Logical.

Here are a few ideas on how to add steps to your day.

- If you take a bus to work, get off the bus a few stops before your usual and walk the rest of the way.
- Park in the far rear of the parking lot at work or at your local mall.

- Take the stairs up to your apartment, or if you're on too high a floor, get off the elevator ten flights before your floor and walk the rest of the way.
- Pace back and forth while waiting for the bus or train, while waiting for meetings to start, or while making phone calls.
- Get up and walk around during commercial breaks while watching TV. This will make the breaks go faster, and you'll put in at least ten minutes of walking time per half-hour show.
- Take an extra trip up and down your stairs just for fun.
- Bring your groceries into your house one bag at a time.
- Use the lavatory in your office that is farthest from your desk.
- Take the dog for a brisk walk. If you don't have a dog, take your neighbor's dog for a walk. And if your neighbor doesn't have a dog, take your neighbor for a walk.

Climb! You'd be amazed how many times you go up and down the stairs in your home. But think how lucky you are if you live in an apartment building. A high-rise is great! Choosing to take the stairs rather than an elevator can get your heart pumping and those endorphins flowing. Climbing stairs burns around twice as many calories as walking, and ten minutes of taking the stairs add up to around 65–100 calories burned.

Garden! Weeding and planting your garden or mowing your lawn all count as moderate activity if your pulse is slightly raised and you feel warm while doing them. Five minutes = 26 calories. Ten minutes = 53 calories. Fifteen minutes = 79 calories.

Jump! Try five to ten minutes of jumping jacks or, even better, jumping rope. (A 150-pound woman can burn 45 calories in one five-minute session.) Jumping rope is good for the heart, bones, flexibility, and coordination. All you need is a rope, a good pair of sneakers, and the necessary space. Depending on the intensity of your workout, skipping rope or jumping jacks will typically burn between 35 and 55 calories in a five-minute session, 70 and 110 in ten minutes, and 105 to 145 calories in fifteen minutes.

Spin! Set up a stationary bike or treadmill in front of your TV and turn on your favorite show. You won't even realize you're working out. Five minutes of moderate cycling will burn around 35 calories, and the same time on the treadmill will burn 30 calories.

EACH OF THESE ACTIVITIES IS HELPFUL IN its own way, but try not to do any of them too close to bedtime.

Around the Neighborhood

Jog! Walk around the block several times while you wait for your child to take a music lesson. As your fitness level improves, add one-minute bursts of jogging to your walks. Moderate walking (at two miles per hour) for five minutes = 14 calories. Ten minutes = 28 calories. Fifteen minutes = 42 calories. Jogging burns 25 calories in five minutes, 50 in ten, and 75 in half an hour.

Dance! Whether you do it at a class or home alone with your headphones on, dancing is great fun and good exercise. If you enjoy what you're doing, you're more likely to stick with it and exceed your five-minute target. I prefer a class because I find exercising with other people is a great way to keep motivated. Five minutes of aerobic dancing burns around 32 calories. Ten minutes = 64 calories. Fifteen minutes = almost 100 calories.

Around the Office

Walk! Use a hands-free phone so you can walk and talk.

Walk over to a colleague with a message, rather than emailing.

Use the bathroom on the floor above yours.

Make your next meeting a walking meeting and brainstorm as you pound the pavement.

Any one of these activities can help you to burn 17 calories in five minutes.

Trek! If you have to drive to your appointment, you don't have to miss out on exercise altogether. When you park, leave the car as far away as practical from your destination and walk the rest of the way. If you're shopping, leave your car in the space farthest from the shops, and you'll benefit from the added bonus of carrying your bags back to the car. You will burn around 17 calories for every five minutes of brisk walking, and more if you're carrying heavy bags.

Twenty-to-Thirty-Minute Workouts

Stretch with Resistance Bands

Stretching exercises stimulate receptors in the nervous system that decrease the production of stress hormones. Stretching exercises also relax tight, tense muscles and increase blood flow to the muscles. Stretching increases your flexibility, which helps with balance, so you feel stronger, safer, and calmer.

You can purchase a rubber or latex stretch band at moderate expense at most sporting goods stores. Stretch to your level of comfort; the stretches should feel good. Hold each stretch for at least fifteen seconds and repeat each stretch as time permits.

Hamstring Stretch

Lie on the floor and loop the band around your right foot, grabbing on to the band to create tension. Straighten your right leg as much as you comfortably can while keeping your left leg slightly bent but on the floor. Gently pull your right leg toward you, stretching the back of the leg. Hold for fifteen to thirty seconds and switch sides. As you pull the right leg toward you, keep the left foot on the floor. Repeat, stretching the opposite foot.

Inner Thigh Stretch

Lie on the floor and loop the band around your right foot, holding both ends of the band in your right hand to create tension. Gently lower your right leg out to the side and toward the floor until you feel a stretch in the inner thigh. Hold for fifteen to thirty seconds and switch sides.

Quad Stretch

Sit on the floor with your right leg straight out in front of you and your left leg bent behind you. Lean to the right on your right forearm and grab on to the top of your right foot with your left hand. This will stretch your right hamstring. To stretch your left quad, gently pull your left heel toward your glutes to stretch the front of your thigh. Hold for fifteen to thirty seconds and repeat on the other side.

Side Stretch

In a cross-legged or seated position, hold on to one side of the band with your left hand and reach your arm toward the right. Grab the other end with your right hand and gently pull, creating tension and stretching the left side of your waist. Hold for fifteen to thirty seconds and repeat on the other side.

Chest Stretch

In a cross-legged or seated position, hold the band with a wider-than-shoulder-width grip up over your head. Gently pull your arms out and down as low as you can to stretch your chest. If you have shoulder problems, you may want to skip this exercise.

Upper Back Stretch

Sit on the floor with your legs extended and loop the band around both feet. Cross the band and grab on to each end with both hands close to your feet. Gently curl your back, stretching it toward the back of the room and using the band to create tension and add to the stretch. Keep your abs contracted and try not to collapse over your legs. Hold for fifteen to thirty seconds.

Hip Stretch

Lie on the floor and loop the band around your right foot, grabbing on to the ends with your left hand. Straighten your left leg out on the floor and gently lower your right leg across your body and to the left as low as you can go, feeling a stretch in the right hip and glute. Hold for fifteen to thirty seconds and switch sides.

Exercise Ball

The exercise ball is used to enhance stability, strength, and particularly balance. Like resistance bands, exercise balls are available in most sporting goods stores and are not a major investment. Although this workout is for beginners, if you've never tried it before, you might at first feel unstable. You'll get better as you go. If you need to, sit next to a wall or chair to use for balance.

1. Sit on the ball with your spine straight and place your hands on either side of your hips for balance. Slowly begin to roll your hips in a clockwise circle, beginning with small circles and moving to larger ones as you become more comfortable. Do ten to twenty circles clockwise and then an equal number counterclockwise.

2. Sit on the ball with your spine straight. Hold in your abdominal muscles as best you can. Lift your right foot and then the left in a marching pattern. Start by lifting your feet only inches from the floor and, as you feel more comfortable, lift your knees higher and march faster. Repeat for one to two minutes.

3. Sit on the ball with your spine straight and abs in. Place your hands on the ball or in your lap and lift your right foot off the floor, holding it in the air for five or more seconds as you slowly straighten and raise your leg out in front of you. Lower and repeat on the other side. Repeat five to ten times.

4. Sit on the ball with your spine straight and place your hands on either side of your hips for balance. Contract your abs and slowly walk your feet forward as you slide your body down onto the ball. Start by walking forward only a few steps at a time, until you feel more comfortable. Continue walking your feet forward until you're in a bridge position with your head and shoulders supported by the ball, hips lifted. Now walk your feet all the way back until you're seated again and repeat three to five times.

5. Stand against a wall with the ball propped behind your lower-mid back. Walk your feet out a bit so that you're leaning against the ball, feet about hip-distance apart. Bend your knees and lower into a

squat, rolling your back down the wall. Go as low as you can but no lower than ninety degrees, which means your thighs are parallel to the floor. Your knees should remain over your toes as you roll down into a squat. Push through your heels to come back up and repeat fifteen times.

6. Lie flat on the floor with your heels propped on the ball. Keeping your abs tight, slowly lift your hips off the floor (squeezing your buttocks) until your body is like a plank, in a straight line. Hold for a few seconds and lower, repeating ten to fifteen times. To make it easier, place the ball under your knees rather than under your heels. To make it harder, cross your arms over your chest.

When You Have an Hour or More

If you have an hour or more—lucky you!—try any of the following:

- Take any class that moves you around, such as dance, yoga, tai chi, sailing, golfing, or belly dancing.
- Join a softball, Frisbee, hockey, basketball, or soccer team or group.
- Go to a batting cage and hit baseballs.
- Go to a driving range and hit golf balls.
- Play tennis, handball, or racquetball.
- Hike in the woods or on a nature preserve.

FULL-BODY WORKOUT

VENUE CHOICE

If time and/or location is not an issue, and if you want to do some full-body work, here is a series of exercises that work well for me.

BELLY

Floor Crunch

Lie on the floor with your back flat, hands behind your head, knees together, feet flat on floor.

Roll your shoulders up as high as you can, keeping your knees stationary and elbows out.

Lower slowly to the ground, one vertebra at a time.

Do three sets of twelve reps.

Leg Extensions

From a back-lying position, sit up a bit, keeping your arms bent on the floor behind you for support. Balance on your buttocks with your legs extended in the air a few inches off the ground. Contract your abs and bring your legs in over your belly bending your knees as you do so. Straighten your legs and repeat.

Do two sets of fifteen reps.

Oblique Abs

Lie on your back, knees bent, feet flat on the floor, hands locked behind your head, elbows out. Roll up until your shoulder blades are off the ground and twist your right elbow toward your left knee. Count to three. Lower and repeat on the other side.

Do three sets of fifteen reps.

LEGS AND BUTTOCKS

Leg Raises

Lie on your back, legs straight out, feet flexed. Lift your legs together as high as you can without lifting the small of your back off the floor. Lower and repeat.

Do three sets of twenty reps.

Lunges

From a standing position, step forward with your right leg so that your thigh is parallel to the floor and your knee is over your ankle. Bend your left knee, lowering your hips until your left knee is about two to three inches from the ground. Stand back up and repeat with the left leg.

Do two sets of twenty lunges.

Donkey Kick

Get onto your hands and knees. Lift one leg up as if to kick the ceiling with the flat bottom of your foot, and lower. Repeat twenty times with each leg. Do three sets.

UPPER BODY

Push-Ups

Go into a full push-up position, with legs extended behind you, elbows bent and close to your body. Lower yourself to the floor, nose pointing down, head even with the rest of the body.

Do ten reps, then rest sixty seconds. Repeat two times.

Plank

Lie on your right side with your elbow on the floor under your right shoulder. Extend your leg in line with your heel. Hold for thirty seconds. Repeat on left side. Do three sets.

STRETCH ROUTINE

Without stretching, the body loses flexibility. The good news is that stretching is not at all hard. Bonus: You'll see your flexibility improve even if you stretch only once a week. As a rule of thumb, each stretch should be held for the following time periods:

Beginner: up to ten or twelve seconds

Intermediate: fifteen to twenty seconds

Advanced: more than twenty seconds

You should never feel any pain with any of these stretches. If you feel pain, stop immediately. The next time you begin, be more gentle with your movements and work your way slowly up to the full stretch.

Neck

Stand up with your arms resting comfortably by your sides. Let your head drop forward. Then slowly roll your head from side to side in a wide circle. Do this two times clockwise, then reverse the motion.

Chest

Stand with your back against the wall. Place your upper arms out to the side, parallel to your shoulders, elbows bent with fingers pointing to the ceiling (like a tree trunk and branches). Your shoulder blades should be touching the wall. Try to remain as flat against the wall as possible.

Upper Back

Sit in a chair with your knees bent, feet flat on the floor. Place your hands on your knees. Bring your chin to your chest and arch your back outward. Continue arching until you feel a stretch in your spine and between your shoulder blades.

Lower Back

Lie on your back with one leg outstretched and the other bent to your chest. Grasp under your knee (at the back of your thigh) and gently pull your knee to your chest until you feel a light stretch in your lower back. Repeat with the opposite side.

Hip Flexors

Stand with one leg forward and one leg back in a lunge position. Allow your back heel to come up and your back knee to bend toward the ground. Let your pelvis tilt up until you feel the stretch.

Hamstring/Calf

Find a step and place both feet on it. Support your weight with the front half of the soles of your feet, and let your heels hang over the step. Rock gently up and down for several minutes, keeping your balance.

Buttocks Stretch

Lie on your back with your knees bent at ninety degrees, and place your right ankle on your left knee. Pull your left knee toward your chest until you feel a stretch in your right buttock. Support the position by placing your hands behind the left knee. Repeat on the opposite side.

AT THIS POINT, I'm going to assume that you are well on your way toward sleeping better, and that having done some of the exercises we have just discussed, you're also moving better. You should know that as you continue to progress, using these exercises through the four-week program, things will continue to improve.

So now you're ready for tool number five, which will teach you how to view the world through a confident, optimistic, and positive lens.

Aren't you feeling better already?

CHAPTER SIX

Mind over SuperStress

WE ARE ONCE AGAIN ENTERING THE REALM OF THE MIND. But whereas in Chapter 3 we explored tools that summon relaxation by resting the mind, we are now going to explore ways in which we put our minds to work to lessen the burdens of SuperStress. The mind is more than just a vessel of thought; given the right directive, it can be a powerful healing agent, too.

You actually can teach your brain how to change the way it views the world, in much the same way that a good pair of glasses can change your vision. Think about what happens when you go to the ophthalmologist: you read the eye chart (or at least you try) and if it's fuzzy, the doctor keeps trying different lenses until eventually the letters come into perfect focus. In this chapter, I'm going to show you how to adjust your own perceptual lenses until the world looks much more manageable. And you're going to make that adjustment using nothing more than your thoughts.

I consider optimism, positivity, and resilience the *primary colors of living well* and I believe that all of them are in our power to embrace. I am not a psychologist, but I have found these ideas to be extremely useful in the ways I treat patients who are suffering from SuperStress. In the four-week program, you will be asked to implement these tools of the mind in varying ways, as assigned homework. And as you do, you'll take a giant step toward transforming yourself and your lifestyle. Let's examine each of them separately and see why they have such power over SuperStress.

OPTIMISM

Optimism is thinking Chicken Little was wrong and the Little Engine That Could was right.

Optimism is cashing your weekly paycheck and dropping part of it on a lottery ticket.

Optimism is running for president of just about anything.

Optimism is investing in the stock market.

Optimism is planning an outdoor wedding in the spring.

In short, optimism is the expectation that good things will happen in the future. When you're optimistic you see possibilities, not problems; you easily weather an adverse situation because you see it as temporary. You have hope.

In his book *Optimism: The Biology of Hope,* Lionel Tiger, a sociologist from Rutgers University, offers an evolutionary explanation for the existence of optimism.[1] Tiger explains that it was biologically essential for our ancestors to be optimistic: if early man believed every undertaking was more likely to end up in disaster than success he never would have taken up the challenge in the first place. So it stands to reason that rather than heading out in the driving rain in search of food for his family, a guy might be inclined to sit around the cave all day. Well, we all know that didn't happen—with the cavemen who survived, anyway. So what sent our man, spear in hand, out into the cold and rain? My guess is that it was the very same thing that sends modern man onto the golf course despite ominous weather reports: optimism.

The Benefits of Optimism

Nothing erodes our belief systems like stress. As we noted earlier, Super-Stressed people have three overarching beliefs:

1. They believe that they're not stressed.
2. They believe that they don't have enough time for everything they need to get done.
3. They believe there is no way out of the time-crunch bind. That is, they have no hope.

If you can change all three of those beliefs, you'll take a giant step toward increasing your optimism and reducing your SuperStress. To begin with if you're SuperStressed, you must recognize that you are. Take a step back and ask yourself if you're suffering from some physical malady that you can't control—a bad back or migraine headaches or irritable bowel or any stress-related health problem. Then you need to ask yourself how you ended up in such bad shape. Were there any circumstances that coincided with the development of this ailment, such as a catastrophic event, a difficult relationship, a toxic workplace environment, or an inordinate amount of work?

Once you get to the underpinnings of what put you in this state in the first place, then you need to ask yourself: If I could change something, would that change mitigate my physical problems? That may be hard to answer. Sometimes only time will tell, and only if you put the question to the test. Can you make the change you have in mind? If you haven't done so already, go back to Chapter 2 and fill out the questionnaires. Seeing the results in black and white might help crystallize the answer for you.

GRANTED, THERE ARE PLENTY OF EXTERNAL STRESSORS THAT WE CAN'T CHANGE. The bills aren't going to stop coming. If you're a working parent, you're always going to be pressed for time, and your family will always need more of your attention. Maybe your fiancé just called off the wedding; maybe he's taken up with your best friend. Maybe there are days when you feel isolated, or betrayed, or overwhelmed. But I'm here to tell you that in the end, you'll have more control over your life and you'll feel far more hopeful if you don't buy into the negativity.

How is optimism going to help? Well, for starters you're taking a mental stand against the notion that there is no hope. Optimists are nothing if not hopeful. Next, you're going to be healthier, happier and more pleasant to be around. You'll worry less. And you'll also live longer. Who doesn't want to embrace all the life they can?

Scientists learned serendipitously about the physical benefits of optimism in the mid-thirties, when the William T. Grant Foundation decided to follow a group of healthy men throughout their entire adult lives in order to learn which specific lifestyle factors determined success and good health.[2] Participants were selected from five separate fresh-man classes at Harvard. All the men were healthy, smart, and socially adept, but they varied greatly in their socioeconomic backgrounds. Based on essays they completed (shortly after returning from World War II) the students were characterized as optimistic or pessimistic. At the start of the study, and then every five years afterward, the men received physical checkups, were interviewed, and answered question-naires about their lives. The results surprised even the investigators. They showed that being born with a silver spoon in your mouth didn't predict life success or health nearly as well as optimism did. Optimists were on the whole far healthier than the students whose early essays revealed more pessimistic attitudes. The pessimistic men came down with diseases of middle age earlier than the optimistic men, and by age forty-five the overall difference in the health of the two groups was significant. In fact, beginning at age forty-five and for the next twenty years, optimism stood out as one of the primary determinants of good health.

Another famous and often cited study began years ago as a longitudinal study of 180 Catholic nuns. Handwritten autobiographies from each of the nuns, composed when they were an average age of twenty-two, were scored for emotional content; researchers then tracked these women through the rest of their lives.[3] As with the Harvard study, when all the data was in, researchers discovered an outcome they weren't expecting. They found that the nuns who were optimistic in their twenties and thirties lived as much as ten years longer than those with neutral or pessimistic outlooks.

Lest you think that a small group of nuns isn't exactly a representative sampling of the population, here's another major study: the Georgia Centenarian Study was conducted between 1988 and 2006, and involved a group of men and women who had all passed their hundredth birthday, meaning they'd already lived twenty years longer than the average American.[4] But these were not frail individuals quietly living out the end of their days. To the contrary, 20 to 25 percent of these centenarians were still living in their communities, mentally intact and generally vibrant. The investigators wondered what specific biological, psychological, and sociological characteristics fueled these long lives.

They examined a number of traits associated with extreme longevity: status, personality, coping strategies, and even diet. And indeed, all these did play a role. But the most important trait—shared by nearly all the centenarians—was a strong sense of optimism.

Rather than focusing on the hard times (the majority of those in the study had been poor all their lives), they chose to remember the good ones. Rather than concentrating on what they didn't have, they concentrated on what they did. Of the ninety-six people in the study, 86 percent were women and more than half of them were African American, a subset of the population that in the past century has not had the easiest of lives. But what they did have they greatly appreciated: the family and friends they were blessed to share their lives with meant far more to them than the stuff by which so many of us measure our happiness.

The four most common traits among the Georgia centenarians were all characteristics we identify as measures for managing Super-Stress.

- Optimism
- Sense of purpose
- Engagement in multiple activities
- Resilience

Can We Become More Optimistic?

Optimism *can* be learned. The concept of "learned optimism" had its inception back in 1964, when Martin Seligman—now considered the father of Positive Psychology but then a twenty-one-year-old University of Pennsylvania graduate student—and his colleagues began work on a laboratory experiment in an effort to better understand animal behavior. The young men placed a number of dogs in a confined space and exposed them to a series of random, uncomfortable stimuli from which the animals soon learned they could not escape. After repeated attempts the dogs began to accept their fate. A short time later, the same dogs were put in an environment where they could escape the stimuli if they chose to. And yet, only some did. Others remained as they had been, passively enduring the discomfort. These dogs had essentially learned to be helpless. Seligman went on to successfully apply this concept of learned helplessness to certain types of depression in people, theorizing that—just like the dogs—some people who feel beset with problems have stopped believing they can do anything to improve their situation.

All the time he was working on the theory of learned helplessness, Seligman wondered about the dogs that moved to safety. Why had some jumped at the chance to escape but not all? Was the same true for people? Why do some people overcome negative circumstances while others are apparently stuck in their role as victims? And more important, if people could learn helplessness, could they also *unlearn* it?

Perhaps, he considered, there was a way, without years of therapy or drugs, to teach depressed human beings how to thrive and flourish in the world around them. Eventually he came up with this idea: to be your happiest, you should not look at what's wrong and needs fixing, but rather focus on what's right and try to make it even better. This remains the principle behind Positive Psychology, a discipline that gave rise to the study of happiness as a science, which seems to have taken hold not only in this country but throughout the world.

So, can optimism be learned? The answer is a resounding *yes*!

The How-tos of Optimism

If being optimistic is your goal—and why wouldn't it be?—there are some things that you can easily do. Well, perhaps it won't always be easy, but work at some of these suggestions and they will come more easily as you go.

1. When you find yourself faced with a problem, stop, consider your options, pick one or two, and just barrel ahead with those solutions. If you think you can, you can.
2. The minute a pessimistic thought enters your head, recognize it for what it is and quickly replace it with a positive one. Take a walk in nature and look at all the good in the world. You can crowd out any bleak thoughts by merely appreciating the beauty around you.

3. Clean house. No, not in a literal sense. What I mean is, to the extent that you can, avoid people who drain your energy by judging you, belittling you, or burdening you with their problems. Who needs people like that when you're looking at life on the bright side?

4. Role-play. Act as if things are just great and your actions will fast become a self-fulfilling prophecy. Optimistic people move faster, talk faster, and project an upbeat attitude. When someone asks how you are, tell them you're terrific! Even if you can't do this sincerely all the time, try it today. And try it tomorrow. You'll soon believe it, too.

SEEING LIFE'S PROMISE: THE POWER OF POSITIVITY

Some people have all the luck. They seem able to maintain a relatively positive attitude despite circumstances that would make you want to scream. They see the good in difficult people and they see opportunity in a challenging situation. In short: they see possibilities. When you become SuperStressed, your luck changes. Because of the negative physical changes and the surging cortisol, you're likely overflowing with negativity, feeling isolated, and hunkered down against the weight of the world; perhaps you now expect the worst. Lacking hope for a simpler, saner pace of life, you've let your inner critic run wild and you may be making poor choices because you feel fundamentally unsupported. And it's a vicious cycle, a hard pattern to break: all those negative emotions keep you bogged down, triggering a flood of yet more damaging stress hormones.

Because positive emotions keep the sympathetic and parasympathetic nervous systems in balance, you need to be in a positive emotional state for as much or more of the time than you are in a negative state to keep SuperStress at bay. Positivity—which I often interchange with the term "positive attitude"—and optimism are related but distinct mental attributes. Optimists believe they are accountable for good things that have happened to them and that more good things are headed their way. If something bad happens, optimists tend to write it off as an isolated incident, an anomaly, or something out of their control. Positivity, on the other hand, is a lens through which we view our daily affairs. With a positive attitude you see the bright side of life and expect good things to come your way. People with a positive attitude wait until they have the facts before jumping to negative conclusions. For example, when your boss leaves a "please come see me" note on your desk, you can conclude that layoffs are in the works and you're on your way out. Or you can believe she's checking on the status of the big project you're managing and would much prefer to hear you talk it through than read a long, involved email with spreadsheet attached. I'm not suggesting that you ignore your intuition or your ability to interpret cues—because sometimes that note *will* bring bad news, even if not a layoff—but don't dismiss the possibility that an ambiguous message could be a good one. In this case, you have to go in to see that boss anyway. Why not arrive on her doorstep with the expectation that you are needed instead of that you are not? That kind of expectation breeds positivity: when layoffs come, you might not be the person to go because the office just can't live without your sunny disposition.

How to Develop a Positive Attitude

Cliché alert! Yes, we're talking here about making lemonade out of lemons. For people in the SuperStressed state, the first step toward developing a positive attitude is to recognize that you feel hopeless. Step two is to understand that you can *change* that feeling.

According to Barbara Fredrickson, author of the book *Positivity,* if we entertain several positive beliefs every day, we'll go from 10 percent feeling good about ourselves to 90 percent a lot faster than you might think.[5] Fredrickson cites many components to positivity—joy, gratitude, serenity, hope, pride, amusement, inspiration, and awe. In her book, she explains that we should try to incorporate these ways of thinking into our lives, and that, she says, is because *thinking makes it so*. I say reach beyond thinking to experience. Go for the brass ring! Grab yourself those positive experiences, and not just once in a while. As those positive experiences become habitual, you'll create a powerful biochemical change in your body. The result: you will have generated your own antidote to SuperStress! (How's that for positivity?)

Crossing the Great Divide

As with optimism and pessimism, there are many ways to cross over from negative to positive thinking. Here are some I've had the most success with:

1. Laugh: The Power of Ha!

One of the things I marveled at when I first went to Micronesia was how many jokes people told in the course of a conversation, often in the course of conversations where a joke was the last thing I expected to hear. For instance, there were always jokes and laughter at funerals. It wasn't that people were belittling the person who had died, or that they weren't sad. Rather, it was the islanders' way of lovingly coping with emotional pain. They were celebrating all that was good about that person's life and, indeed, his or her death. That experience taught me that you can feel something that's sad or painful but you can still have hope, you can still look forward to the future.

Laughter is a great way to blow off steam in any society, but I find that Americans are more inhibited about laughter than most traditional cultures. We don't start out that way, though. From the first smile at about six weeks, babies start to laugh and then spend increasing amounts of their day laughing. By age six, the average child laughs three hundred times a day.[6] Unfortunately, though, the laugh meter peaks at six. A seven-year-old is likely to curtail his or her merriment in deference to social training or peer pressure. You know what I mean. When someone trips, a five-year-old will laugh, but by the time that child is ten, he may think it's funny, but he knows it's not socially acceptable to laugh. And so it goes, until a person reaches adulthood, and the laugh meter bottoms out at a paltry fifteen to one hundred chuckles a day.

This is unfortunate, because it turns out that laughter is quite healthy for us. Dr. Michael Miller and other researchers at the University of Maryland School of Medicine in Baltimore have shown a direct link between laughter and healthy function of blood vessels.[7] Laughter appears to cause the tissue that forms the inner lining of blood vessels to expand in order to increase blood flow. Using emotionally provocative movies to gauge the effect of emotions on cardiovascular health, Dr. Miller and his colleagues studied a group of volunteers whose mean age was thirty-three. Each volunteer was shown part of two movies at the extreme ends of the emotional spectrum: the opening scene of *Saving Private Ryan* and of *Kingpin*. They saw the beginning of one movie on one day and two days later, the other. Overall, average blood flow increased 22 percent during the funny movie (*Kingpin*, in case there was any doubt), and decreased 35 percent during *Saving Private Ryan*.

2. Lose the Negative Self-Talk

We all talk to ourselves all day long. Even when our lips are motionless, we're hearing our own voices and they pass judgment on our every move. Many of us live with the constant chatter of a harsh inner critic that guilt-trips us about things we have said or done and makes us doubt whether we're good enough at anything. When you believe such negative self-talk, you may perceive things as more stressful than they actually are. For example, when you tell yourself something is frightening—such as giving a speech—it becomes more stressful to deal with than if you tell yourself that saying a few words in front of a dozen colleagues who trust your judgment is a challenge you can easily surmount.

Not all of our inner voices are negative. Sometimes they affirm how good we are by telling us what we've done right. The problem is, we rarely pay much attention to our inner cheerleader. Say you're hiking up a mountain on a glorious summer day. Do you think of how lucky you are that you're experiencing no joint pain? No. Do you compliment your feet for supporting your trek? Of course not. But let one tiny little blister develop, and you're on your own case for the rest of the day. You should have worn hiking boots. You should have brought a Band-Aid. You should have done something about the pebble in your shoe when you first felt it chafing. It seems that it's always what we do wrong that gets our own attention. Not what we do right.

Can you silence your inner critic? It's certainly worth a try. Putting a stop to negative thoughts and nurturing positive internal dialogue can reduce stress and empower you. You can start by appreciating some of the good things around you. When you're furious at yourself for getting lost despite the "foolproof" directions at hand, look out at the landscape and enjoy it for its novelty. Savor the experience. You've probably learned something along the way (to bring a map, for starters . . .).

You also might try repeating some of the affirmations from Chapter 3. Whatever your choice, understand that if your goal is to change your behavior, it's more effective to stop telling yourself negative things than just to tell yourself positive things. It's not so much the power of positive thinking as it is the power of nonnegative thinking.

3. Cultivate a Sense of Gratitude

Gratitude is so much more than just saying "thank you" for a gift or a benefit received. Gratitude is taking the time to acknowledge that you are truly grateful for something (or someone) that has entered your life; that you feel lucky, even privileged, to have had that event happen to you. For our purposes, gratitude is a perfect antidote to negative emotions because you can't be both grateful and miserable at the same time. The brain cannot process a positive and a negative at the same time. You can't be happy *and* sad, brazen *and* shy. So if you're SuperStressed, and you want to get on with your life, cultivate a sense of gratitude.

One of the best ways to cultivate gratitude is to keep a gratitude journal, which combines the benefits of journaling with the adoption of a more positive mind-set. You'll be instructed how to do this in the four-week program. In the end you'll have a catalog of happy memories to look back on every time you need to remember how lucky you are.

In her book *The How of Happiness*, psychologist Sonja Lyubomirsky of the University of California at Riverside, suggests keeping a daily diary in which you write down things for which you are thankful.[8] She suggests you choose a time of day when you have several minutes to step outside of life and reflect. Consider three to five things you are grateful for, from the mundane (you found your misplaced cell phone, your husband brought you flowers) to the magnificent (your child's first steps, the beauty of the sky at night). Think, too, about the people who care for you and those who have touched your life. Lyubomirsky has scientifically studied the results of taking the time to conscientiously count blessings once a week for a period of six weeks. The subjects of her study significantly increased their overall satisfaction with life, whereas a control group that did not keep journals had no such gain.

At the University of California at Davis, psychologist Robert Emmons found that engaging in gratitude exercises—that is, *directly expressing* gratitude to someone to whom you are grateful—elevated mood, raised energy levels, and, for those who suffered from certain ailments, helped to relieve pain and fatigue.[9] You'll see in the four-week program that I have suggested you take a few minutes every so often to call up a friend and say "thank you"—if only for being your friend. You'll be amazed how good it makes you feel.

RESILIENCE

Who hasn't taken an arrow to the heart from which you were certain you'd never recover? At some time or another, all of us will encounter relationship problems, health issues, financial stresses, job concerns, and loss. This is life. But here's the central question: When confronted with a thorny situation, how do you respond? Do you face the challenge head on? Or do you look for the nearest rock to hide under? In the face of adversity, do you bounce back or do you land with a five-pointed *splat*? If you're among the SuperStressed, you may not exactly *splat,* but my guess is that you're not going to bounce very far, either.

One powerful way to increase your resilience is to recognize and acknowledge the beliefs you hold that are derailing your attempts at happiness. A second is to play to your strengths. Let's look first at the belief factor.

Iceberg Beliefs

In their book *The Resilience Factor: 7 Keys to Finding Your Inner Strength and Overcoming Life's Hurdles,* Drs. Karen Reivich and Andrew Shatte identify one of the barriers to resiliency as what they call "iceberg beliefs."[10] We all, they write, have deeply held beliefs that sometimes lie so far beneath the surface of consciousness that we're not even aware of them—or at least, we refuse to acknowledge them. Which can make them difficult to identify. Though these beliefs operate at an unconscious level, they still have the power to chip away at our resilience and relationships.

Sam and Jamie's Story

To show you what I mean, let's look at a suburban married couple. This couple happens to be hypothetical, but they bear a close resemblance to many couples I have known. Sam, the husband, a TV producer, commutes from Connecticut to New York and often gets home at ten at night. He leaves at seven in the morning, which doesn't allow much time for sleep. When he's sleep deprived, he's not always the nicest person.

His wife—let's call her Jamie—has her own full-time job selling real estate in their hometown. She works hard at her job, too, but because she's at home more and is the one in charge of the house and the children, she does the lion's share of the housework. When they moved from the city to the suburbs, Sam and Jamie made a deal. She would take care of the day-to-day running of the house, and he had only one task: to put the garbage cans at the foot of the driveway for pickup twice a week. But often when he gets home, it's late and he's tired; he's stressed and preoccupied. For whatever reason, he forgets—or just doesn't do it.

So one fine garbage pickup day, Jamie is in the kitchen by the window, sipping her first cup of coffee when she notices that the garbage truck has passed her house without even slowing down. Furious, but knowing all too well what to expect, she charges into the garage to find that the cans are still there, filled to the brim, and beginning to smell. Sam comes down for breakfast, and the first thing Jamie does is jump on him. They have a huge fight in front of their six-year-old son. This is not the first time that he's forgotten to do it, it's the *tenth* time! she yells, and he counters with a "So what? I didn't do it! Can you just get over it?" Jamie perceives his behavior as disrespectful. Plus, he's gone back on his end of the bargain. So she kicks up the volume a few notches—and he storms off to work feeling lousy.

Are they fighting about garbage? Of course not. The garbage is only the tip of the iceberg. The iceberg is made up of beliefs they both subconsciously cling to, and as a result it is causing them both stress. She has some unspoken anger at him and he has some unspoken anxiety with which he can't cope.

What Sam needed to do was ask himself why it was such a problem to honor the deal he and his wife had made. Why (for the tenth time) didn't he put the garbage by the curb? If he dug down deep, he would realize that he perceives the take-out-the-garbage duty as the last in a long line of duties in his day. He meets hundreds of demands a day at work and he comes home to more. And he hates it. If Jamie dug down deep, she would see that what she's feeling is that she's not getting enough respect from Sam.

In their entrenched and negative (stressed) states, both have defaulted to behaviors that give them no positive feedback. Because he didn't own up to the fact that he wasn't coping, Sam defaulted to a choice that was not useful—he walked away. Jamie, on the other hand, just fought harder. They both unconsciously chose behaviors that made them feel worse and worse and worse. In this situation, the couple had reached a grim deadlock from which there was no bouncing back. What they could have done brings me to a second, surefire way to incorporate resilience into your life. And that is, to lead from your strengths.

Leading from Your Strengths

Some people who are reeling from an unexpected crisis or are struggling with a difficult relationship blame themselves for the mess they're in. Like Martin Seligman's helpless dogs, they lie down and tell themselves that's just how it is. Others try to fix what they think they're doing wrong. Recall that positive psychologists consider trying to fix what's wrong a colossal waste of time. It's far better, they believe, to look for what you do *right* and try to do it even better, to identify what you do best and let those capabilities—positive psychologists call them "strengths"—steer you through life.

Everyone has strengths. They are the abilities, assets, virtues, and qualities that you excel at and that give you joy. Your strengths might include such things as hope, playfulness, bravery, valor, curiosity, love of learning, good judgment, integrity, and emotional intelligence.

> You can identify your personal strengths by taking a free test developed by Christopher Peterson, professor of Psychology at the University of Michigan, which can be accessed on the website www.authentichappiness.com. The test takes around thirty minutes to complete and measures twenty-four character strengths that have been valued across time and cultures. It gives you a ranking of your character strengths from the strongest to the weakest. Your top strengths are considered your signature strengths. Once you know what they are, you can summon them to help you become more resilient when dealing with hard times. Even when times are good, try to find ways to use one or more of your signature strengths every day.

Let's say our couple Sam and Jamie heeded this advice. Here's what might have happened: Since he is a TV producer, you might not be surprised to hear that Sam is decisive, fair, and gets things done. Unrelated to his work, he also possesses a deep love of family. Using those strengths, he sat down with Jamie and explained on the spot exactly what he was feeling, from being overwhelmed with work to being tired when he got home and wanting nothing more than to have dinner and relax. He then suggested a compromise: if she would take on the responsibility for the garbage, he would take the children by himself one afternoon every weekend, so that she could enjoy some well-earned time for herself. Jamie's strengths are her artistic talent, her love of learning, and her engaging personality. Love of family is also one of her signature strengths. She accepted Sam's compromise because she believed it would be wonderful for the children to have an afternoon with their father, and because she could now spend that alone time painting with oils—something she had been dreaming about having the time to do since the children were born.

That Sam and Jamie—two deeply SuperStressed people—could compromise on a situation that had earlier seemed hopeless to both of them, and from that compromise move on to a far better relationship, says much about how to use your strengths to summon resilience.

THE ART OF COPING

Here's the given: We know we're stressed, even if we haven't yet acknowledged our SuperStress. We know, too, that we can't change our stress-laden environment. But we *can* change how we respond to that environment, and that's what I mean by coping. I use the word *art* judiciously, but I really do believe that there is an art to how one copes with SuperStress. The way you cope reflects whether you are handling a situation well; and whether you are feeling overwhelmed. It also can help you understand whether you have arrived at the right balance.

Numbing and Dumbing

Unfortunately, many SuperStressed people cope in ways that compound, rather than fix, the problem. Their strategies may temporarily reduce stress, but they cause more damage in the long run. They use nicotine, alcohol, and drugs (prescription or otherwise) as a means of dealing with anxiety. The rate of substance abuse in those with post-traumatic stress disorder runs four times higher than in the general population, and, though it has not been scientifically proven, I believe from seeing patients in my practice that many SuperStress sufferers replicate this pattern.

While users all seek the same result—to feel better—nicotine, alcohol, and recreational drugs operate through different physiological mechanisms. For example, smokers believe that they need cigarettes to relax, but in fact nicotine is a stimulant with zero sedative effects. In a study that provided tobacco to both nonsmokers and nicotine-craving smokers, only the smokers reported that it improved their mood. Nonsmokers given nicotine generally became anxious and irritable.

A typical cigarette contains about 6 to 11 mg of nicotine, with 1 to 3 mg going directly into the smoker's bloodstream. From there it goes to the brain, where nicotine triggers the release of dopamine, a neurotransmitter linked to feeling pleasure. With each puff of smoke, the brain gets an instant reward, which explains why cigarettes are so addictive. When smokers try to quit, they experience levels of stress significantly higher than those of nonsmokers. However, the good news is that if they can scale that initial hurdle, smokers who quit become less, rather than more, stressed. More important, they greatly improve their odds of reaching their senior years.

Alcohol numbs the brain. Is it any wonder that people who want to escape their problems raise a glass or five? The brain can detect an infusion of alcohol within minutes of consumption and responds by altering the balance of the neurochemicals glutamate, gamma-Aminobutyric acid (GABA), dopamine, serotonin, and the opioids. Alcohol increases dopamine, opioids, and serotonin, easing anxiety and promoting a sense of well-being. Animals, birds, and even butterflies are naturally drawn to intoxicants, so it's no surprise that humans would be too. But for people who are SuperStressed, alcohol can be seductive. It holds out—and fulfills—the promise of quick relief, but can only ever be a temporary solution.

The third category in this trifecta is drugs. Opiates can relieve pain without causing unconsciousness and create a sense of dreamy deep relaxation in the user. All humans are naturally dependent on opioids for emotional health. Both narcotics and our natural endogenous endorphins act by bonding to specific receptors and neurons in the brain and scattered along the spine. Narcotics also trigger dopamine release, which heightens the sensation of well-being and is one reason they're so highly addictive. Of course, none of these problems arise with the body's natural, endogenous opioids, which are the biochemical building blocks of serenity. People with SuperStress who have been prescribed such opiates for physical pain are especially vulnerable to getting hooked on them.

In addition to smoking and self-medicating with alcohol or drugs, some people use sleeping pills or tranquilizers in an effort to mediate their SuperStress symptoms. Others overeat, oversleep, go on sexual benders, or fill up every minute of their day so that they don't have to think about what's really bothering them. They're afraid to plumb their emotional depths—afraid of what they'll find there.

Remember the three beliefs of SuperStressed people: they don't believe they're stressed, they feel like they're chronically out of time and they have no hope for a change anytime soon. When my patient Leanne first came to see me, she knew she was stressed, but she continued to subscribe to the other two beliefs. Her lack of time to "get everything done" overwhelmed her, and she saw no way out. She arrived at my office looking for ideas on how to cope with her stress.

Leanne's Story

Leanne had two sets of twins—eight-year-old and eleven-year-old boys. Each of the four children played a different after-school sport on a different team, and someone needed to shuttle them all to practices and games on almost a daily basis. Problem number one: there was one driver—Leanne. Problem number two: our wife/mother/driver was unbearably overworked because she had more obligations than hours in her day. Problem number three: she believed she had to find a way to do it all—and do it by herself.

Leanne thought she had to be supermom because she grew up in a family where her mother was a high-powered, self-sufficient lawyer who was highly competent, though she never had to deal with twins (she only had Leanne and her brother, Patrick). Dinner was never late, the kids never missed a birthday party, and she always had (or made) the time to talk through a problem or help Leanne and Pat with their homework. Because Leanne had such respect and admiration for her mother, she patterned herself after her. And even though her neighbors considered Leanne the most competent wife and mother on the block, their awe did nothing to alleviate her stress. For the past six months she had been waking up at three in the morning wracked with anxiety, and recently her hair had started to fall out.

I asked her what her time management options were. "I have no options," she told me. "I need to get all this done and I'm the only one who can do it."

"But it doesn't look like you're making any inroads," I said. "I gave you sleeping pills that aren't working. Your muscles still hurt and your hair is still thinning. Don't you think we should be thinking of something else?" There was, after all, *some* help available to her. Her mother was nearby and willing to pitch in. And Leanne's husband was more than willing to pick the boys up after games. But she didn't want to give up any of her responsibilities. To do so was to admit she was less than a perfect wife and mother. I explained to her that there is no such thing as a perfect wife or mother, and that with a growing list of physical problems, she was running out of time. "The more sleepless nights you spend, the more you erode your resilience," I said. I learned later that when she awoke at three, she considered it the perfect time to go downstairs and do the laundry!

After another month of watching her hair get thinner and the circles beneath her eyes grow darker, Leanne gave in. Together, we made a plan to simplify her life. We agreed that she would join at least a couple of carpools, attend fewer of the children's games, allow her mother to come in to help on Thursdays, order pizza on Wednesday night, and accept more help from her husband. I told her to come back in a month. She did and, much to my dismay, still looked exhausted. That was when I realized that the stress was taking over her life. If we were to have any success, we had to dig deeper. It wasn't enough to remove some of the obstacles in her way. Leanne had started doing less for her family, but she still wasn't doing anything for herself.

On her next visit, we began to identify what she could do that might help her feel more in balance. Together we decided she needed two things: more time for herself and a weekly date night with her husband. It wasn't that he didn't value her. He did. He wanted to help, but she never let him. Leanne's circumstance was another iceberg situation— iceberg beliefs also include ideas about how the world should operate and how we should operate in the world.

The tip of the iceberg for Leanne was how she was going to get the kids to the game. But what was beneath the surface was her need to really be valued. She felt humiliated because she wasn't perfect. She felt like a failure because she didn't live up to an idealized version of what *she* thought she should be. She lacked self-awareness of what was at the bottom of her discomfort. I sent her for talk therapy and she was able to dig down emotionally to see what was eroding her chance for happiness. Once she understood herself better, she was able to relinquish the unreachable standards she had set for herself and to relax. The more she learned to appreciate her strengths rather than try to fix her weaknesses, the better she was able to sleep. After several months, her hair stopped falling out.

Some of the best ways to cope are right in front of our noses, if only we choose to recognize them. Knowing yourself and what you want is one way of coping with SuperStress—provided, of course, that you act on that knowledge. But another approach involves reaching outward.

Jordan's Story

My patient Jordan is almost a poster child for how strong positivity and optimism can truly change difficult situations for the better. Were it not for Jordan's extreme determination and optimism he would be in a very different situation than he is today. Jordan is a divorce attorney and marriage mediator who, several years before I met him, began suffering from awful pain caused by a clump of blood vessels (hemangioma) that were compressing part of the spinal nerves in his back. He had the hemangioma surgically removed, but the pain remained. It grew to such a degree that he could not sit even for ten minutes without pain—a terrible fate for an attorney and mediator, whose day involves many hours of sitting immobile in a conference room. Since he was no longer able to do this, Jordan was forced to abandon his beloved profession.

Jordan was referred to me when it seemed that he had tried every medical option, including epidural injections and electric stimulators, to deaden the pain. Nothing had worked. "Having to retire was bad enough," Jordan told me that first afternoon in my office, "but I'm also still in pain!"

He sounded frustrated and defeated. He explained that he was devastated at having to be on such strong narcotic medications because they represented a dependency that made him feel like a victim. I asked him why that was, and he said because it robbed him of his greatest joy: flying. He had been forced to give up his vocation and now, because of their narcotic effects, the pain medications disqualified him from his avocation, too.

What I saw was a man who was understandably depressed and overwhelmed by the blows life had dealt him. But I also saw a man who looked willing to try just about anything. I decided to explore a new avenue, one that took us away from his physical problems: I asked him to tell me more about what flying meant to him.

"It's everything to me, Dr. Lee," he said, adding that he was willing to pursue any avenue for pain relief "if it will put me back in the air."

We talked very candidly about what it might take for him to reclaim that dream. I told him it wasn't going to be easy, but that I thought there was a good chance he could accomplish what he wanted to. As soon as the words were out of my mouth, and for the first time that morning, I saw a small spark of joy reflected in the man's eyes. So we set up a plan. I introduced him to a psychotherapist who taught him self-hypnosis, which he practiced every day. And I got in touch with his pain doctor who started weaning him down from his medications—very, very slowly.

By Jordan's second visit, which was six weeks later, he said he felt a little bit better. He told me he had been religious in devoting at least twenty minutes a day to his mind/body exercises and had never missed a session with the psychotherapist. With his pain doctor's help, he had begun tapering off and had halved one of his medications, with some difficulty but with his eye on the goal. He might have three good days but they would be followed by a bad one when the pain returned. But he was full of optimism. "After all," he said, "three good days! Next time there will be four and then we're on our way." With that attitude, he made me optimistic, too.

It was a rocky course, that first year. Jordan was challenged by episodes of flaring pain and withdrawal symptoms that occurred with each step down from the narcotics, even though the reductions were very small. But he kept up all his treatments and continued to do his mind/body exercises. After a while he began to mentor others in the legal field, and he acknowledged that doing so gave him a purpose. It also, he said, kept him busy until he could be back in the air.

Over the next two years Jordan slowly and methodically, with the help of his pain specialist, continued to reduce his medication. His psychotherapist, a very accomplished hypnotist and mind/body specialist, devised a daily exercise, which helped him visualize himself flying in the near future. We also spent many sessions adding other mind/body exercises to strengthen his visualizations and keep him in touch with his goal. We started adding music as another way to take his mind off pain. He loved symphony music and this was well suited for enhanced relaxation.

By the beginning of the third year, Jordan was finally off all medication and his pain was minimal, often nonexistent. He seemed thrilled with his progress and asked me for a letter requesting a reevaluation of his condition so that he could resume piloting. I sent him for rigorous medical, psychological, and neurological tests—and he passed them all with flying (excuse the pun) colors.

Today Jordan is flying once again. It was a long and difficult road with many moments when the only thing that kept him going was his positive outlook: his belief that he could and would do whatever it took to be able to fly again. But that's not the end of the story. Jordan was so grateful for his success in overcoming adversity that he decided it was time to give back. He began to donate flying time to taking children with cancer, some of whom had never before been in the air, for short airplane rides.

Jordan's story is a great example of how one man's optimism, positivity, and resilience allowed him to experience one of life's greatest gifts. And I'm not referring to being able to go up in an airplane. Rather, I'm speaking of one of the most beautiful ways—and my favorite, given the choice—of diminishing your own challenges: by being able to do something for someone else. And that is what the final two tools in our toolbox are all about.

CHAPTER SEVEN

The Power of Connection

IN THE EPIGRAPH that opens his famous novel *Howards End,* the author E. M. Forster issues this two-word directive: *Only connect.*

Writing about class difference and hypocrisy in early-twentieth-century British society, Forster realized the deep psychological need for connection in humans. The enduring popularity of that 1910 novel shows that he was far from alone in his understanding of this concept. In my own lifetime I have experienced three defining moments that reflect the power of connection and community. Strangely enough, each was linked to a death.

The first occurred during one of my early trips to Micronesia. I treated a patient, an elderly woman named Mary, who was suffering from congestive heart failure. I understood the problem well enough, but without high-tech medical equipment, which was unavailable to me, there was nothing I could medically do for her. Still, as she continued to deteriorate day by day in the hospital, I met and chatted with an ever-growing circle of family members and close friends—feeling wracked by guilt that comfort was all I could offer. After a long hospitalization she went into cardiac arrest and died, and I expected them to blame me for her death. Yet much to my surprise, they embraced me; they were grateful for the respect I had paid her and the family, and were touched and appreciative of my compassion for their loss. In their minds, it was highly unusual for an outsider to spend that much time getting to know not only her but *them.* They welcomed me again at her funeral, which began with a feast followed by an all-night session in which two groups of women took turns singing stories about Mary, her childhood adventures, old loves, funny incidents, and favorite foods and jokes. The songs both celebrated Mary's life and taught the young people of the village about their past. It was a remarkable experience, a rare but beautiful time when caring for a patient heals the doctor.

The second death happened much closer to home: last year I lost my mother. For as long as I can remember, my mother struggled with serious mental illness, and ours was often a difficult relationship. When she suffered a debilitating stroke, I was consumed with regret for all those years I hadn't fully expressed my love *for* her *to* her. I arrived at the hospital hours after hearing that she was gravely ill. My sister, who has always been the strongest member of our family and the one who nurtured my connection to my mother, was already there. Each of us took one of her hands and told her how much she meant to us. A few hours later, she passed away. At the moment of her passing, I saw, for the first time, peace in her eyes.

The third death occurred just a few months ago, and it struck me as painfully emblematic of the twenty-first century. After a long workday, I was dozing on the train ride home, dreaming about the weekend ahead, when suddenly I heard a woman shout, "Is there a doctor on the train? We need a doctor!" I sprang to my feet and saw a man, who looked to be in his late fifties, slumped over in his seat behind me. Five people eased him to the floor so I could start resuscitation. Someone called for an ambulance to meet us at the next stop, and I sent someone else to ask the conductor for a defibrillator, only to learn there wasn't one on the train. I did CPR, but the man quickly went into shock. After we pulled into the station, the waiting paramedics lifted him onto the stretcher, where I watched him die right before my eyes. Strangely, not a single person on the train seemed to know who he was. Not one. Did he have a wife? Partner? Children? If he did, how tragic and yet predictable that in our disconnected society, someone could be so alone and anonymous at the end of life.

The following Monday as I rode to work, I looked around and realized that I had been traveling on that same train between my hometown and Manhattan for *eight years* and yet I knew very few of the people around me. I decided to try to connect with at least some of my fellow passengers. As I turned to the woman next to me, I couldn't stop thinking: that man could just as easily have been me. And nobody would have known who I was.

PEOPLE WHO NEED PEOPLE

People need people. And people who are SuperStressed need others more than most. If you're SuperStressed, you're far more likely to isolate yourself from the world because you're generally so focused on a single goal. Most of the time that singular focus comes at the expense of everything and everyone who could be supportive, who could make you feel loved, appreciated, and valued.

Long ago when I was in training, one of my fellow medical residents—I'll call him Mark—fit squarely into this category. One fine Tuesday, one of the attendings at the hospital asked Mark to present a talk at Grand Rounds, an honor for a resident and one Mark was determined to make the most of. He had only a week to prepare for this talk, so he closed out everything and everyone for that period of time. When he had free time—and residents don't have much—he spent every minute of it researching his subject and preparing slides. His fellow residents, including me, watched in amazement as he became completely absorbed in his task. He hardly slept, he ate nothing that didn't come from a vending machine, and he totally isolated himself from anyone who might have distracted him for a few moments or shared a healthier bite to eat when he desperately needed it. By the time Grand Rounds rolled around, he was nervous, jittery, and a red-eyed physical mess. The talk was fine. Mark, however, was not.

But let's say that he did decide to stop in the hall and have a few pleasant words with a colleague, or that he took a ten-minute coffee break with a friend. That could have made a world of difference for him. Why? Because connecting with others, even for a short time, can completely change your physiology. Connecting with others relaxes you. It tones down your sympathetic nervous system (the fight-or-flight force) and fuels your parasympathetic nervous system (recovery mode). When you're SuperStressed, you're stoking your cortisol machine, and that's no way to live. You can't run forever at top speed—you'll just collapse. You, and any number of your bodily systems, need a rest. Think of the hunter who is being chased by a predator and finally ducks into the safety of his own cave. Stress response; recovery. Overexertion; sigh of relief.

Did Mark breathe a sigh of relief when it was all over? Sure. But he could have gone into that meeting feeling (and looking) a whole lot better if he had blown off some of those pretalk nerves hanging out for a little while with his buddies. More important, he would have recovered faster. Fortunately for Mark, his deadline was clear, and Grand Rounds came and went.

But what if his life was an endless series of Grand Rounds–like pressured goals, demanding all of his time with no room for family or friends? While I can't predict exactly what Mark might face in twenty years in terms of medical problems, I do know that the duration of SuperStress he'd face would provide a welcome mat for any disease he was genetically and environmentally vulnerable to—bumping up the odds that a heart attack or some other major illness would come knocking at his door.

AN AGE-OLD NEED

Many thousands of years ago, with the help of our limbic system, evolutionary biology made it practical—and safe—for humans to live in packs. But despite the continued workings of that very same limbic system, today's groups seem to be fragmenting. Perhaps because we no longer need to fear predators. Or, more likely, we Americans have taken the mission of independence set down by our forefathers in the Constitution to heart. No matter. Social connection in the United States has changed drastically over the past few decades, and the fabric that binds us together is wearing thinner all the time. In our great-grandparents' (and for some of us, our grandparents') days, extended families and villages provided each of their citizens with membership in the community where they lived and worked. In those days, everyone played a role. Older people were respected for their life experience. Teenagers helped look after younger children and children, in turn, helped around the house or on the farm. Automobiles may have been scarce or unknown, but friendships were not. Your neighbors cared for you when you were ill, helped fix your broken sink, and watched out for your children as you did for theirs. On Main Street, the cop waved at the teacher, the doctor asked about your mother's migraines, and scores of people knew who you were and where you belonged. In such small communities, people largely felt safe, cared for, and at home.

ISOLATION NATION

I wish I could say that America is going back to the days when friends and family played a significant role in our lives. But it appears that, if anything, we have become a nation of loners, all but abandoning our close societal bonds. While our distant ancestors lived in stable social groups of two hundred or so, the advent of the global economy has stretched our social units to 6 billion. On a stage the size of our planet, how many of us can say with conviction that there's a place we know we belong?

Our friendships aren't doing much better, either. According to sociologists at Duke University, Americans' circle of confidants has shrunk dramatically in the past two decades, and the number of people who say they have *no one* with whom to discuss important matters has more than doubled.[1] That same study, which compared data from 1985 and 2004, found that the mean number of people with whom Americans can discuss matters important to them dropped by nearly one-third over that fourteen-year period.

In his book *OverSuccess: Healing the American Obsession with Wealth, Fame, Power, and Perfection*, author Jim Rubens cites some equally distressing statistics, such as that spouses in dual-income families with children spend an astonishingly small amount of time talking to each other every day: twelve minutes. The typical American adult now spends nine hours each day—more than any other waking activity—consuming some form of media, which is an isolating and isolated pursuit if there ever was one.[2]

Why is this happening? What went wrong? In this day and age, staying connected is a challenge for many reasons.

Fear of strangers. Many of us are simply afraid to connect. Particularly in large urban areas, we cross paths with hundreds of people every day, but we're taught that making eye contact invites encounters best avoided. Don't encourage strangers, our parents instruct. And we listen. So we end up like that man on the train, surrounded by a clutch of people, knowing none of them.

I recently heard this story about a woman's commute home from her job in Manhattan. She got off the subway at her stop in Brooklyn and as she climbed the stairs to street level, she noticed a man several steps behind her. During the three-block walk to her apartment building, the man stayed close behind her, and he stayed right with her as she unlocked the lobby door, went into the elevator, and even when she got off on the sixth floor. Now, her heart racing, she turned to the left while quickly pulling out her key from her handbag. He turned left, too. As she slid her key into the lock of her front door and started to twist it, the stranger walked past her, took out his keys, and opened the door to the next apartment. It turned out that they had been next-door neighbors for nine years and had never before seen each other.

Though the initial lesson of isolation is obvious, I think the larger lesson is that we don't have to accept leaving things this way. The woman in Brooklyn, through her experience, now has a new awareness of the degree of her isolation and she had an opportunity to get to know her neighbor. I wondered. Did she? Would she? Perhaps, like Seligman's dogs in the experiments with uncomfortable stimuli, she had learned a kind of helplessness about her isolated situation. Unfortunately, I never learned the answers to these questions.

Fear of rejection. You can't strike out if you don't step up to the plate. Some people are more comfortable avoiding connection altogether than putting themselves in a situation where they might be turned down. Nothing is more isolating than isolating yourself by choice. If diving headfirst into a sea of people or crossing a room to make a new friend is not your idea of fun, you might start by following the Japanese philosophy of *Kaizen*, which preaches the power of baby steps. Try joining a group of like-minded people—a knitting group at a local yarn store or a reading group at your local library. This allows you to test the waters without making a major commitment. Baby steps. Works every time.

Geography. People are so busy these days that spontaneously dropping in on a friend is a gesture that has gone the way of the telegram. One of my New York City–working friends told me she only allows herself to socialize with people who are GD.

"GD?" I asked. "What is that?"

"Geographically desirable, " she replied. Which she defined as "living within a twelve-block radius of my apartment." Does anyone bring a cake to the new neighbor anymore? Why bother? If the statistics are to be believed, they're probably going to move sometime in the next three years anyway. Or you are.

Technology. With half the American population digitally savvy, perhaps it should come as no surprise that technology trumps relationships at every turn. According to a recent poll, nearly one in four Americans says that the Internet can serve as a substitute for a significant other for a measurable period of time.[3] That's almost 25 percent of us, everyone! The same poll reports that more than one in four Americans has a social networking profile on a site such as MySpace or Facebook. Among eighteen-to-twenty-four-year-olds, that figure rises to 78 percent. Who says it's hard to make friends? They're only a click away.

And what about our modern-day coffeehouse experience? In the European coffeehouses—of fin de siècle Vienna, people met and sat around drinking coffee as they discussed the political, cultural, and social issues of the day. Does that sound like any chain coffeehouse you've visited lately? Is *anyone* having a conversation with anyone but the folks behind the counter taking orders? Of course not. They get their lattes, stake their claim to a table near an electrical outlet, and set up their laptop for the duration.

While you might find cell phones ubiquitous and annoying, particularly when people use their cellular voices (screaming into their phone in public places), at least those people are talking to someone. With text-messaging, it's flying fingers that do the talking, threatening to relegate real conversations to the same fate as the handwritten letter.

And then there are those pesky handheld games. In the days of yore, when Mom picked up her ten-year-old at school, he'd get into the car and they'd talk about what he did in class that day. Now he climbs into the backseat, clicks his seatbelt, pulls his handheld game from his backpack, and immediately engages with the moving screen. She might ask about his day, but chances are she won't get more than a muffled monosyllabic reply. How can she compete with the increasingly realistic virtual environments that game makers spend millions on?

What is all of this isolation doing to us personally? It is clearly taking a great toll on our individual physical and emotional health. What is it doing to us as a nation? Multiply that toll by 300 million.

THE HIGH COST OF LONELINESS

Loneliness is an emotion we all feel at some time in our lives. But make no mistake: loneliness is not about being alone. You can be alone and not feel lonely at all. Loneliness is a feeling of being isolated even though people may literally surround you. Louise Hawkley, a researcher at the University of Chicago, suggests that loneliness isn't just isolation but may also be closely related to perception. She says lonely people tend to perceive stressful circumstances as threatening rather than challenging, and that stressed, lonely people don't ask for support or try to change what's creating the stressful situation but prefer instead to withdraw. Which keeps them even more isolated. In her 2006 study, she reported that high blood pressure and loneliness were strongly linked, especially in older adults.[4] And we all know that high blood pressure is a forerunner to heart disease.

Scientists have shown that lonely people's blood vessels are less elastic, their hearts are weaker, and their levels of inflammation and stress hormones are higher. Furthermore, loneliness affects the immune system. In a study reported in *Health Psychology* in 2005, Sheldon Cohen, professor of psychology at Carnegie Mellon University, and his colleagues found that first-year college students who had smaller social networks and greater loneliness had worse immune responses to flu vaccine than those students with a more expansive network of friends.[5]

Another study by Cohen's team found that people with the greatest number of social roles and domains of social connection—highly integrated people, in the study parlance—are less likely to smoke and drink in the face of social pressure than those who have fewer social connections.[6]

A study of more than four thousand Californians in Alameda County directly linked their longevity with the size of their social circles. The greater the number of friends, the greater the longevity. Those whose regular contacts were fewer than six had significantly higher rates of blocked coronary arteries. They also were more likely to have diabetes, high blood pressure, and depression.[7] A British study showed that in the first year after a wife dies, her widowed husband has a 40 percent risk of death, and in Europe, research suggests that kissing on a regular basis provides additional oxygen and stimulates the output of antibodies.[8]

The bottom line: connection is essential to good health. Our hearts know this. And, as researchers have shown, our whole cardiovascular and immune systems know it. Now we just need to get it into our heads.

The Connection to Self

SuperStressed people need to make special efforts to connect with others. But of equal or even greater importance is their having and nurturing a connection to themselves. And most don't. Asked to list the most important people in your life, whose names would you put down? Would your own name even be on the list? Asked to write an essay about a friend or family member, you could probably do it easily. But do you know yourself well enough to write about who you are?

Self-relating is one of the most important concepts of psychology. And yet, when I try to talk to my SuperStressed patients about their dreams and desires and the things that inspire them, most don't have much to say. I tell them: if you don't know who you are, you can be sure no one else knows you either. But they still cannot answer.

This is in stark contrast to the people I treat who have their stress under control. They're energized by their dreams and welcome the chance to talk about their desires, because those desires so truly express who they are. The biggest difference between living a meaningful life and living in a Super-Stressed condition is that one perpetuates itself and the other eventually exhausts itself. SuperStressed people are so focused on meeting a goal, on planning for tomorrow and the next day and the next, that they have no energy for anything else. They occasionally connect with others—when it moves them closer to their goal. But they rarely connect with themselves.

It doesn't take a lot to connect with yourself. All it takes is slowing down enough to hear the voice within telling you what you value, what is meaningful to you, and then living your life by those principles. It sounds so easy, but of all the essential elements necessary to reach a genuine SuperStress solution, placing your attention squarely in the here and now is one of the toughest, particularly for those already in a SuperStressed state.

THE IMPORTANCE OF TOUCH

Connecting is not only about relationships; it's also very much about true physical intimacy, human touch. Every living being thrives on touch. Including rabbits.

There's a famous story about a group of atherosclerosis researchers who studied the effects of plaque buildup in the arteries of rabbits, a study that they hoped would one day provide help to humans with coronary artery disease. In the laboratory, rabbits in their individual cages were stacked up in columns that reached almost to the ceiling. Periodically, each rabbit was administered a specific type of cholesterol that would build up over time and eventually narrow their arteries. When it came time to examine the rabbits' arteries the researchers found that rabbits whose cages were in the lower tiers had 60 percent less plaque in their arteries than the ones in the upper tiers. How could that be? All the rabbits were given the exact same dose of cholesterol. So what accounted for the different levels of plaque? The puzzled scientists decided to spend more time in the lab observing the animals directly. They didn't have to wait long before the key to the puzzle revealed itself. It came in the form of a diminutive female lab attendant who loved animals. As she tended to the rabbits, she would warmly stroke the fur of the ones she could reach. The touch made the difference. To confirm this, one of the researchers rearranged the cages so that the rabbits on top also could feel the love. Suddenly, the once touch-deprived animals' health improved, a direct result of the attendant's special attention: the power of touch.

In humans, touch is sometimes a matter of life and death, particularly for infants and the elderly. Children who are adequately fed and cleaned but deprived of all but the barest of human contact will fail to grow at a normal pace. There is even a name for them: failure-to-thrive babies. One isolated case tells of a baby boy who was abandoned on the steps of a New Jersey hospital. Based on his physical size, doctors guessed his age to be somewhere between eleven and fifteen months. He was emaciated, barely moving, and by a cursory study of his legs, the physicians determined he had never stood up or even attempted to crawl. He was placed in the hospital nursery and the doctors, assuming he might be a failure-to-thrive baby, immediately started him on a regimen of TLC. The prescription? Any nurse or aide who had a free hand had to pick up "Spencer" and carry him along on his or her tasks. He received his bottles and food while sitting on the lap of anyone who was available, including the receptionist at the nurses' station. Within weeks, Spencer began to grow. Within six months he had put on twenty-five pounds. A few months after that, he was walking and talking. All the while, the physicians continued to reevaluate his physical age, upping it considerably until they finally determined that the boy who when he was abandoned had the physical dimensions of a one-year-old was, in fact, two and a half years old on the day he was left to the hospital's care.

Failure-to-thrive babies are often found in the orphanages of war-torn countries, where overcrowding keeps them in close quarters but emotionally and physically isolated; many never feel the touch of another human being except when it's absolutely necessary. They're actually worse than "not thriving"; they have lost the will to go on. The depression they suffer diminishes their appetite, so they don't gain weight. Their small bodies generate stress hormones, which elevate their heart rates and depress their growth hormone function, so they stop growing. In institutional care, many simply die. Fortunately, if the babies are removed from the isolating situation and placed in a safe and nurturing environment in due time, as with Spencer, they can recover quickly.

BUILDING A SOCIAL SUPPORT NETWORK 101

So far, this chapter has illustrated the importance of connecting to others and how doing so will protect you from the surging stress hormones that can take a physical toll on your body. But opening yourself to others is not only defensive; it can be good for your health, too. One study demonstrated that close support among women makes them less apt to overeat, more likely to eat well, and less likely to turn to substance abuse, and it stimulates them to exercise.[9] Emphasizing the link between connectedness and resilience, another study showed that patients with larger social networks demonstrated lower perceptions of pain after surgery, used less pain medication, and experienced less postoperative anxiety, particularly in the first five days following surgery.[10]

But perhaps more important, opening yourself to others will also add new meaning to your life—on many levels. First, having a network of friends can increase your sense of self-worth. Having friends means that others value you—your ideas, your sense of humor, your lasagna Bolognese. They enjoy something about you and the things you do together. Why else would they be your friends? Second, connecting with a group, or even a single friend, provides a sense of belonging and helps ward off loneliness. If you stop at the local deli in Quechee, Vermont, on just about any morning, you'll see a group of men having coffee together. They call themselves the ROMEOs, which stands for Retired Old Men Eating Out. These not-so-young men have been known to brave roads covered with winter ice and snow and sub-zero temperatures just to spend that hour with one another. Such is the power of a social support system.

But how can you create one for yourself?

A social support system is comprised of friends, family, and peers. It's easier to build than you might think. One tried and true approach is simply to spend time with those whose company you genuinely enjoy. We're talking quality here, not necessarily quantity. People seem to get more joy from spending longer periods of time with a close friend, rather than running around amongst a bevy of buddies, according to researcher Meliksah Demir, Ph.D., assistant professor of psychology at Northern Arizona University.[11] One of the essential pleasures of close friendship, Demir found, is simple companionship—or, as he puts it, "just hangin' out" one on one. If you have a group of friends, nurture the relationships by staying in touch, being proactive (call your friend for a cup of coffee; don't wait or stand on ceremony regarding who called whom last), being a good listener, and taking time to appreciate your friends and letting them know that you do.

Some more ways to be a friend include learning to laugh at yourself, facing the world with hope, finding a confidant with whom you can share your dreams and disappointments, and being a confidant to someone else.

If your social circle is smaller than you'd like, I have two words for you: *get involved*. In any way you can, from being a hands-on grandparent to joining a neighborhood committee to volunteering in any one of a thousand ways. If you decide to volunteer, choose a cause that's important to you. In that way, you'll meet others who share your values, which makes the connection stronger from the beginning.

WHEN RELATIONSHIPS GO BAD

Bear in mind that the goal of extending your social support network is to mitigate your stress level, not add to it. So it's essential to recognize and be wary of relationships that lead you *away* from your goal. I'm referring to what I call "toxic relationships."

All relationships inherently include two people, and the give and take of any liaison opens the possibility that we may lose a piece of who we are. If the relationship is worth the investment—if you're receiving as much as you give—consider yourself lucky. But what if the relationship is not worth it? What if it is not a give-and-take relationship, but rather a give-and-give? And give. And you're the giver.

Why would you stay? Why does anyone?

People remain in bad relationships and endure abuses for many reasons, not the least of which is fear. They stay because they're afraid of being alone or because they're afraid to leave, erroneously believing that the devil they know is better than the devil they don't. Some stay in abusive relationships because they feel that they deserve it. What they perhaps fail to consider is the serious impact such relationships have on their health and happiness. In addition to piling a mountain of anxiety and stress on a person, a bad relationship destroys their self-confidence and makes them isolate themselves from well-meaning friends and family.

I see this most commonly in marriages where one or both members of the couple are miserable, and yet they stay together for their children, or because they have a new house or major debt, or for any number of reasons, sometimes just to preserve their image as a happily married couple. The problems compound when, even after choosing to remain a couple, they make no effort to mitigate or resolve their situation. They never attempt to change their conduct. That's because they've become emotionally numb to the toll their unhappy relationship is taking on their health. Because they can't feel the pain, they remain in a state of limbo, telling themselves and others that everything is fine. Because they think that it is. Sometimes people forget that they have a human birthright to feel joy and pleasure.

Toxic relationships aren't confined to domestic couples, by the way. They can be found between work colleagues and even the closest of friends. You might have a dear childhood friend who has always been like a sister to you but who, as you've grown older, has become increasingly difficult. In deference to your history together, and because you hate hassles, you always give in to her. If you think about it, you might even say that if you were meeting her for the first time today you wouldn't try to make friends—that's how much she has changed. Still, you keep her around. Why? Perhaps you truly love her. And that's fine. But what's not fine is that you haven't spoken up about what's bothering you. That's not real love. If you love somebody, but your relationship is now one that saps the love right out of you, find a way to talk to that person. That's what a relationship is all about. It's not going to be an easy conversation, but it must be an honest one.

THE GOOD NEWS

The message to take away from this chapter is that people simply cannot live a meaningful or happy life without including, in some way, other people. For all of us, and particularly for the SuperStressed, it is critical that we be committed to family and friends and continue our efforts to keep these ties strong. The good news is: you are entirely in control of your own situation. It's up to you. You can choose how you want to connect and with whom, and you can decide how much of yourself you want to invest in building social connections.

The most important way to connect, I have always felt, is reaching out in service to others. This should come as no surprise considering the profession I chose. Given the opportunity to name the one person who influenced my choice, I would name my grandfather, whom I lived with in his plant-filled apartment off and on from the time I was eight years old. He truly knew the power of connection. My grandfather was a first-generation Chinese American who came from China to live in San Francisco, where he ran a restaurant and then a laundry, occupations that always kept him in service to others. I stood by his side as he shared himself with his family and his community, which, he reminded me, was an honor and a privilege. Whenever anyone he knew fell ill, my grandfather made his special soup (the recipe can be found on page 264), and I was given the job of walking with my grandmother to that person's home to deliver it. This was no small feat for either of us, as the neighborhood presented some very steep hills. From apartment to apartment we would go, dropping off soup, exchanging news, and offering hopes that the recipients would soon recover. I suppose I missed the significance of it, because I recall becoming impatient after a while. But in retrospect, I believe that those trips played a larger role in shaping my future than I gave them credit for. Today, thanks to my grandfather, I recognize the importance of connection as one of the master keys to a resilient life. And it often costs no more than an investment of your time and perhaps a jar of soup.

In any case, the results are priceless.

CHAPTER EIGHT

The Life of the Spirit

LONG BEFORE I ENTERED THE FIELD OF MEDICINE, Dr. Bernard S. Siegel, then a surgeon at Cornell University Medical School, began a journey of self-exploration. His goal was to deliver the highest-quality medical care and to help people heal. But despite many triumphs, he felt that at some fundamental level he was a failure; something was missing—particularly when it came to treating people with terminal conditions. He decided to put the question to patients directly: "What more can I do for you?" Their answers surprised him, to say the least. Rather than entreating him to find a miraculous cure, they asked for something beyond medical expertise. Something, he thought, a minister or rabbi might be better able to provide.

What his patients wanted was to be *cared for;* to find a path, perhaps outside the confines of what conventional medicine could do, to self-healing and self-love. Siegel heard this over and over from people with all kinds of diseases and from all walks of life until he realized that what was missing from his ministrations was a spiritual component. Of course, none of these patients presumed that a spiritual physician would cure their disease in circumstances where others couldn't. It was that these people wanted to *keep living*—not just to stay alive. They wanted to experience and grow despite the limitations set by their disease. And they wanted their doctors to be their partners in this quest. Most people still have this desire, but unfortunately, the delivery of modern health care has conspired against fulfilling it.

With the advent of HMOs in the 1970s, medicine became and still remains first and foremost about the bottom line. These days, many physicians barely fulfill their role as healers. It's not that we don't value our patients' hopes and desires. We do. But because of the economic pressures that have crept into the way doctors treat patients, we're so pressed for time that conversations about spiritual development are near the bottom of our priority list, following histories and physicals and tests and lab reports and test results and prescriptions and forms and more forms.

I wish those who set the terms of how we practice understood the importance of a rich spiritual life: that a lab report never held a sick person's hand; that an MRI, for all the essential information it provides, will never answer the question: *Why did this happen to me?* Those ministrations require real people with real voices. Doctors are those people. We took an oath to treat a person, not a disease. And yet, with the scores of patients we see in a day and the short amount of time allotted to each, we barely have a chance to learn their names. The idea that we'll have time to care for a patient's spiritual needs is all but a dream.

Which is why this chapter is so important. If you want to find—or reconnect to—your spirit, I hope this chapter will answer some of your questions or at the very least help you start that spiritual journey. It will assist you in laying the groundwork for discussions with your physician, your priest, your rabbi, your parents, your grandparent, or anyone you trust and love. Finding your spiritual self will help you deal with some of the hardships you are facing and relieve the SuperStress that attends them.

Spirituality is not religion. Religions are institutions with rules and regulations. Religions incorporate public rituals and organized doctrines, while spirituality is a private, personal experience. At its core, spirituality gives context to our lives. It serves as the internal compass that orients us to the world beyond our selves. Spirituality arises from connections with yourself and with others, as well as from your personal value system and your search for meaning. For some, this takes the form of prayer, meditation, or a belief in a higher power. For others, it can be found in time-outs from our daily chores, moments when we appreciate music or art or find the time to take a walk in the woods. Spirituality provides the sense that we are part of a greater whole.

AN ANTIDOTE TO SUPERSTRESS

SuperStress sufferers are often in such a state of spiritual crisis that they've lost the feeling that a unique light shines within them. Because they are so fixated on getting through any given day, putting things into perspective is difficult if not completely foreign to them. When I ask my SuperStressed patients what's meaningful to them, many react as if I'm out of my mind. They're so overtaxed and depleted that they regard a conversation about "meaningful things" as a very low priority. They remind me that they have a long list of other goals—getting out a report before the next morning, or finding the right dress for a daughter's wedding, or, for that matter, finding their misplaced keys in time to pick the kids up from school. None of these stressors is long-term, but as a group they can become chronic. Life should not be about making a to-do list and adding two new items every time one is crossed off.

Research shows that people who are more religious or spiritual use their spirituality to cope with life. They're better able to cope with stress, they heal faster from illness, and they experience increased benefits to their health and well-being.

Research also tells us that people who are spiritual have far less stress in their lives than those who are not. This makes perfect sense to me, because spiritual people understand the importance of letting things go. To illustrate the power of this simple but significant concept, I often use the following exercise with my patients: I hand them a small stone, about the size of a golf ball, and tell them, "Stand up and hold your arm out straight in front of you, palm down. Take the rock in your outstretched hand and squeeze it hard, as if you're going to crush it into powder." The tighter they squeeze the more they restrict blood flow into their hand. Soon it starts to be uncomfortable. After another minute or so I say, "Now open your hand and let the rock fall to the floor. What do you feel?" What they feel, what they *always* feel, is relief. "Well," I explain, "that's what letting go feels like."

But spirituality is not only an antidote to what ails you. It does much, much more. On an intellectual level, spirituality connects you to the world, which in turn enables you to stop trying to control things all by yourself. When you feel part of a greater whole, it's easy to understand that you aren't responsible for everything that happens in life.

- One study of nearly 126,000 people who are actively involved in their religions (a meta-analysis of the results of forty-two individual studies) found that those who frequently attended services increased their odds of living longer by 29 percent.[1] The researchers determined that the relationship was so strong it would take 1,418 new studies showing no association between religious involvement and living longer to overturn the significance of the findings.
- A study by the National Institute for Health Research (NIHR) showed that Canadian college students who were connected in some way with campus ministries visited doctors and medical clinics less and had less stress during difficult times. Those students who had a strong religious connection also showed higher positive feelings, lower levels of depression, and were better at handling stress.[2]
- Still another study reported that individuals with an intrinsic religious orientation, that is, those who dedicate their lives to God or a "higher power," are less physiologically reactive to stress than those with an extrinsic religious orientation (people who use religion as means to an end, such as making friends or increasing community social standing.)[3]

The Meaning of Meaning

No two people will ever have identical definitions of what is meaningful. But for me, the definition of meaning is simple and can be summed up in two words: Viktor Frankl.

Viktor Emil Frankl, M.D., an Austrian-born psychologist, was thirty-seven years old in 1942 when, because they were Jewish, he, his wife, and his parents were deported to the Theresienstadt concentration camp. Family members were separated from one another on arrival. Two years later, Frankl was transported to Auschwitz and then Dachau. After he was liberated he learned that the Nazis had murdered his entire family except his sister, who had earlier immigrated to Australia. Frankl wrote the book *Man's Search for Meaning* about his time in the camps. He described how, when he could no longer endure the reality of his day-to-day existence, he found a way out by dwelling in the spiritual domain.

Every day, Frankl wrote, he stood at the barbed-wire fence that kept the starving prisoners captive and gazed through it to a place where, just inches away, he could see a small yellow flower growing in the dirt. Frankl found meaning in that flower. That single bloom helped him focus on something beautiful in a place where horrific and heinous crimes overwhelmed everyone else. What Frankl had that so many other prisoners didn't was the ability to see beyond the fence, beyond that moment to a future that could be better. That future gave him a reason to continue living. He concluded that even in the most absurd, painful, and dehumanizing situation, life has meaning—because there is the hope of moving beyond that situation. Frankl was liberated from Dachau in 1945 and went on to become a world-renowned psychologist. More than fifty years later, he died peacefully in his bed, of old age, in Vienna.

The moral? Everything has meaning. A flower, a baby's laugh, even an automobile accident. Meaning in life surrounds us. We need only go looking for it.

The Meaning of Values

My father used to say: "Never judge a human being by what he says. Look at what he does." While I paid little attention to him at the time, I now understand what he meant. He was referring to a person's values and how they guide a person's actions every day of his life. Values nurture the spirit and inspire a sense of humility and perspective on one's place in the world. You are, after all, a part of the hugely complex interconnected web of humanity. Even if you're famous and wealthy and gorgeous and gifted, you're also a human being. And one of your responsibilities as a human being is to make life better for others. Believing that is a value.

Self-acceptance is another value. Accepting yourself means looking in the mirror and being proud of who you are. Why is this so difficult for so many? Because in this day and age, it doesn't behoove corporate advertisers to reinforce or even acknowledge that you might be terrific in every significant way. To do so would leave them no improvements worth selling and would put them and their clients right out of business. Instead, advertising fuels the demand for millions of products that claim they will make us better, faster, slimmer, prettier, sexier, and yes, even happier. But the truth is that advertisers aren't doing you any favors. Their bottom line relies on you questioning your own self-worth.

When someone tells me that they're low on self-esteem, my first thoughts are: *Well, what do you value? What do you stand for? What do you believe in? What is sacred to you? What would you sacrifice for?* The fact that you would sacrifice for your children and some of your best friends says that you value your family and friends. Beyond this, however, SuperStressed people often don't know what they value or if they themselves are valued. Often *they* don't value themselves at all. As a result, they turn into followers, doing what everyone else is in an effort to be accepted.

Don't do it.

You are giving up every iota of control over your life if you believe that following others' lead is the path to self-worth. Followers are driven by an innate fear that goes back to our ancestors' days: the fear of being banned from the group. You've seen it. Spend a few minutes in the cafeteria of any middle school in any town across the country and you will, in no time at all, identify the "queen bee" and the "wannabes."[4] The queen struts across the school yard and down the halls with a knowing, regal assurance. The wannabes slavishly dress the way the queen dresses and follow in her footsteps. Are they happy to tag along in such a demeaning way? They certainly think they are! After all, they're in with the in crowd. A wannabe is one kind of SuperStressed woman (or man) in the making. As too many adults know, it's not just teens that fear being left out.

Entertaining that fear of abandonment is not only stressful; it leaves people vulnerable to some pretty abnormal-for-them behaviors. I saw this fear in the eyes of Karen, a young woman who breezed through college and then, for no apparent reason, lost herself.

Karen's Story

Keeping up with payments on college loans was such a huge burden on Karen's modest wages that she was obliged to move back home with her parents shortly after graduating. She worked at a variety of jobs, none of which lasted very long. In between jobs, she hung around the house, growing weepy and depressed, regularly numbing her pain with pasta. She gained weight, eventually ballooning to two hundred pounds, at which point she refused to go out at all. She was caught in a downward spiral of shame. The more she ate the more she hated herself, and the more she clung to her self-imposed isolation. And what else is there to do on your own but eat? Here was a woman who was completely SuperStressed, but unlike most in that state, she knew it. She just didn't know how to break the pattern of behavior. Her mother, a patient of mine for years, sent her daughter to me for a consult.

"All my friends are getting married or settled in careers," Karen told me, sobbing. "I just seem to be running in place—like Alice in Wonderland. I can't get a good a job, and I've gotten so fat that my clothes don't fit. And what guy would ever want to go out with me?"

I immediately started her on a weight-loss regimen. That was the easy part. I recommended talk therapy to help her bring her life into focus. But getting her to talk to me about what she really wanted had me stymied. That's because she didn't have a clue. At our second meeting I tried a new tack. "Tell me something, Karen," I said. "What gives you pleasure? If you had to name a person, place, or thing that excites you or makes you feel good, what or who would that be?"

She didn't hesitate for even a second.

"Food," she said, half laughing, half crying.

"Food?" I wasn't expecting that at all. "*Food?*" I asked again. This was going to be much harder than I had thought.

"Yes," she said, nodding. Then she added hastily, "Not so much eating it, Dr. Lee—although you'd never know it now—but working with it. I love to cook for other people. And I'm good at it! My friends love it when I cook. I can always count on making people happy when I cook something. But I haven't done it in ages." Her voice trailed off.

"I don't see my friends too much these days. They all have jobs or families and not much time for me. . . ."

I pondered for a bit, aware that she was looking expectantly in my direction.

Karen said she loved food, but at first glance it seemed that food was what we needed to get her away from. But then suddenly it hit me. Rather than distract her from temptation, I thought, why not put temptation to work for her?

"Okay," I said, "you love to cook? Then what about cooking school?"

She laughed at the absurdity of my suggestion. But then her tears stopped. I could almost see her turning the idea over in her mind. She was quiet for a minute or two, then she looked at me wide-eyed and said, "That's perfect! I can do something I love and something for other people at the same time."

I don't always hit a home run, but I did that day. When Karen left my office, there was a new light in her eyes. Inspiration was written all over her face. In the following months, as we worked together on her weight-loss program, she enrolled in a well-known culinary school in Vermont. She excelled there. In fact she thrived to such a degree that she no longer needed to come to see me. A year later, her mother proudly brought me up to date on Karen's life. After cooking school, she got a job at a Vermont restaurant specializing in regional and seasonal cuisine. When its principal chef left, Karen took over the kitchen and made the place a popular local and tourist destination. The weekend I drove up there to see how she was doing the place was packed.

Karen was slim and lovely as she came out to greet her guests and to introduce me to her fiancé, an organic farmer who was dedicated to sustainable agriculture. What a testament to the power of finding meaning and caring for yourself!

Like many SuperStress sufferers, Karen needed to cultivate enough self-love to access and then fulfill her true needs. Before, she had judged herself by other people's standards, which left her feeling overwhelmed and ungrounded. Her experience illustrates that if we don't have a clear sense of our values we can feel as if we're in freefall, without the power to manage our lives or the resources to combat SuperStress. Her story also showcases the power of getting in better touch with ourselves. Once she was able to understand what mattered to her, she could also right herself and come out of that freefall.

NEW VALUES FOR A NEW CENTURY

In the last century, many of us held materialistic values and many segments of American culture promoted fierce competition and jockeying for power. But if we're to successfully cope with the demands of the twenty-first century, those values must evolve and center on easily ignored ideas, such as developing our spiritual lives and giving back to others.

In the table below you'll see the distinction between the value systems that I've observed in my SuperStressed patients and those who are managing their stress. Much of this difference was a gradual shift that came as we explored what was really important to them. Embracing one or a group of SuperStress values (as seen in the left-hand column) often leads to a life of discontent. But as you start making choices to shift toward the column on the right, you will find that not only do you have an easier time in almost everything you do and aspire to, but that in living this way, your expectations—indeed, your whole existence— are both simpler and far more sustainable.

SUPERSTRESS VALUES	SUPERSTRESS *SOLUTION* VALUES
Respect, Popularity	Self-acceptance
Wealth	Sufficiency
Fame and power	Humility
Showplace home	Comfortable refuge
Perfect spouse and kids	Loving relationships
Striving, overly driven	Loving what you do
Independence, self-determination	Community

Building a Spiritual Path

Can we develop spirituality? Absolutely. Is there a blueprint to follow? Not really. But that's a good thing, because it means that you can go at your own pace and in your own way. What you'll find below is a list of suggestions for ways to become more spiritual. Some might be easier than others for you—after all, each of us is different—but all can illuminate the way to find meaning in your life.

Altruism

In Fyodor Dostoyevsky's great novel *The Brothers Karamazov*, Father Zosima advises his people to "Go help someone. Reach out to a brother or sister in need. Feed the hungry, heal the sick—and then, only then, will you come to know that the world is trustworthy and God is real."[5]

Physician Albert Schweitzer weighed in with a similar message when he said, "One thing I know: the only ones among you who will be really happy are those who will have sought and found how to serve." Today there are so many ways to put these two inspired messages into action. Altruism is the act of giving of oneself out of a genuine concern for others. Not only does it make us feel good to give, it's also among the healthiest things we can do for ourselves. Mom wasn't wrong when she said, "It's better to give than to receive." But I wonder if she understood the full health benefits.

Allan Luks, M.D., who has performed many studies on the positive effects of altruism on human health, worked with more than 3,000 volunteers to establish that after performing an act of kindness, people first feel a rush of euphoria that's followed by a long period of tranquility and well-being. During this stress-reduced period, immune system responses are improved. An incredible 95 percent of his altruistic volunteers enjoyed better health than others of the same age. Studies conducted by other scientists have confirmed the following results, first noted by Luks.

- Helping others contributes to the maintenance of one's own good health, and can diminish the effect of diseases and disorders both serious and minor, psychological and physical.
- Acts of altruism increase self-esteem while producing a feeling of happiness.
- Helping can enhance our feelings of joyfulness, emotional resilience, and vigor, and can reduce the unhealthy sense of isolation.
- The health benefits and sense of well-being return for hours or even days whenever the people recall lending someone else a hand.[6]

Forgiveness

Forgiveness is essential to our spiritual nature because it allows us to release past hurts and failures from our minds. Joan Borysenko, a psychologist, author, and director of a spiritual mentoring program, calls forgiveness "accepting the core of every human being as the same as yourself and giving them the gift of not judging them."[7] In essence, forgiveness isn't so much about letting the other guy off the hook as it is about letting *you* off the hook. When you forgive, you are no longer a victim of your own perceptions. You can change those perceptions: *you do have that choice.* In forgiving, you let go of resentment, anger, hostility, and guilt, all attitudes that directly fuel SuperStress. By forgiving, you protect your own physical self from the flood of damaging chemicals like adrenaline, noradrenalin, and cortisol that attend the stress response.

But forgiving others isn't the only important issue. Sometimes we need to forgive ourselves, and often that is a far more difficult thing to do. Say you made a mistake that cost you dearly. Perhaps you invested heavily in stocks the day before the market took a five-hundred-point nosedive, or you gossiped about your best friend and word got back to her. Do either of these examples sound remotely familiar? Of course they do. After all, who among us hasn't acted rashly or made a bad decision every so often?

How long can you blame yourself for your shortcomings and mistakes? And, in the end, what good does it do you not to let go of the blame? Self-blame only compounds the injury, not just because you're wasting time and energy hating yourself, but because you're also initiating a cascade of damaging stress hormones on top of the bad feelings.

If you're in the midst of a supergrudge against yourself or anyone else, I have three words for you: *let it go*. Like the rocks I give my patients to squeeze—just let it go. Follow nature's lead, because nature is all about healing and forgiving. Dan Custer, in his book *The Miracle of Mind Power*, explains:

> Should you cut your hand with a sharp knife, the forces of nature set about immediately to repair the damage. It was a mistake to cut your hand, but nature does not withhold the repairing of the world. Nature immediately forgives and starts at once to make repairs.[8]

If nature can be that forgiving, why can't you?

Prayer

Prayer is an excellent defense against SuperStress. Through its connection to a higher power, prayer evokes a relaxation response that quells stress, quiets the body, and promotes healing. Prayer also provides feelings of calm, safety, and groundedness. The meditative aspect of prayer produces mental states that induce the relaxation response, thereby lowering pulse and blood pressure and enhancing immunity. Religious people give and receive community support through prayer groups and church socials, so the connection factor comes into play. But understand that you don't need to go to church or pray in an organized, recognizable way to reap these benefits. Praying to your own vision of God or even simply meditating on your idea of God can bring these responses out, too.

Dr. Andrew Newberg is a professor and scientist at the University of Pennsylvania who has researched the neurophysiological correlates of meditation, prayer, and brain function. In an interview, Dr. Newberg explains that "specific practices that have traditionally been associated with religious and spiritual contexts may also be very useful from a mainstream, secular, health point of view, beyond those contexts."[9] Dr. Newberg's laboratory has conducted a study where fifteen older adults with memory problems practiced Kirtan Kriya meditation for a period of eight weeks. The results show very promising preliminary outcomes in terms of the impact on brain function.

For the past thirty years, Harvard scientist Herbert Benson, M.D.—known as the father of the relaxation response—has conducted studies on prayer. He primarily focuses on meditation but he is interested in all forms of prayer because of its ability to allay stress and promote healing. Benson has shown through MRI scans on Buddhists how the brain is affected by prayer. As an individual goes deeper into a meditative state, the brain's parietal lobe circuits—the circuits that establish distinctions between the self and the outside world—are activated, promoting a slowing of brain activity. At the same time, the frontal and temporal lobe circuits, which track time and create self-awareness, become disengaged and the limbic system becomes activated. The result is a sense of awe and quiet. The body becomes more relaxed and physiological activity including heart rate, breathing, and pulse, becomes more evenly regulated. The subject becomes calmer.[10]

But, says Harold Koenig, M.D., associate professor of medicine and psychiatry at Duke University, prayer is not only about slowing down and finding peace. It does far more. His book, *Handbook of Religion and Health,* reviews nearly 1,200 studies examining the effects of prayer on health.[11] These studies show that religious people tend to live healthier lives in part because they're less likely to smoke, drink, or drink and drive. In fact, says Koenig, people who pray tend to get sick less often, as separate studies conducted at Duke, Dartmouth, and Yale universities show. He also notes the following:

- Hospitalized people who never attended church have an average stay of three times longer than people who attend regularly.
- Heart patients were fourteen times more likely to die following surgery if they did not practice a religion.
- Elderly people who never or rarely attended church had a stroke rate double that of people who attended regularly.

• People who are more religious tend to become depressed less often. When they do become depressed, they recover more quickly.

Connection with Nature

Nature is in essence spiritual. Nature lifts the spirits and calms every one of our senses. We respond to the colors of nature on a subconscious level. We know from research that greens and blues have an enormously peaceful effect on us. Nature's sounds soothe us, too. Think of the sound of a babbling brook or a rushing waterfall or birds calling to one another from adjacent trees. Think about the silence of nature, the peaceful quiet of falling snow, a quiet that brings a soothing effect to your nervous system. Take a walk in the woods after a rainfall and inhale the fresh smells: the earthy dampness of the leaves and the fresh scent of pine needles underfoot. Even if you live or work in an urban locale, you will rarely have to go very far to find nature's handiwork. It's in the flower beds in your local park or the flowerpots on the front stoop of your building. Even on a busy city street, you can stop for a few moments and look up at the clouds. These small patches of beauty are sometimes all it takes to remind us of nature's majesty.

Nature is bigger than we are. It gives us perspective and lets us know that while we're sometimes overwhelmed by work deadlines, piles of laundry, or a month's worth of unopened mail, the hassles of daily living are really quite small compared to the ocean and the sky. No matter what happens to us, the mountains will still be the mountains and the rivers will still run downstream.

Experiencing Poetry

SuperStressed people are always getting ahead of themselves. They can be sitting in Carnegie Hall, listening to Yo-Yo Ma play the most extraordinary cello concerto, and spend half the time thinking about what they haven't done or should be doing. Or consider what's going on inside the mind of a SuperStressed woman on a cruise. She's sitting on a deck chair on the balcony of her stateroom, with a tray of crumpets and a pot of tea set on the table beside her. As she gazes out to sea, her eyes adjust to the sun as it begins to slip below the horizon. That's what she sees. But what she's thinking is: *Did I call to break my dentist appointment before I left? I hope the dogsitter isn't overfeeding Rex. What should I wear to dinner tonight?* I call this "mind chatter." It's the incessant noise that comes from fearing what you haven't done or, worse, what you *have* done, but not perfectly.

Where does poetry fit in here? Poems can be a gateway to inner dialogue. At some point in our lives we need time to just think and dream—to let our thoughts rise like bubbles and grant us greater insight into our selves and life in general. Poems lead to that kind of thinking because they leave so much open to interpretation. In almost every indigenous religion, practitioners are given intellectual riddles as part of the self-inquiry process. In some Zen Buddhist practices these are known as koans and they are almost always in the form of short poems. Koans aren't meant to be solved—and can't really be. One fun exercise might be to find two poems that ask you to consider life's mysteries. As you read them, let your imagination wander out of its Super-Stressed state into a world of peace, letting your curiosity guide you in observing how your mind wanders with these ponderings.

An Exercise in Self-Awareness

I share the following four questions to help you follow a thread deeper into your self that can connect you to the things that personally matter most. Before you start, get a pencil and paper to record your answers. Do it now. Then one week from now, do the same exercise and see if your answers have changed. Then try it again in a month.

- If you were ninety-nine years old and looking back, in what ways would you be satisfied (and dissatisfied) with the direction your life has taken?
- What nonmaterial gifts have you received that made you happy? What nonmaterial gifts did you provide that made others happy?
- What gives you joy?
- What part of yourself or your life would you like to leave behind to let the world know you were here?

KINDNESS WILL FIND YOU

Every so often, if she's very lucky, a writer will find a story that sums up the essence of the chapter she's currently crafting. The following story is just right for this chapter on spirituality, because it illustrates how taking a small leap of faith can carry us through the most difficult times, and how trust guides our hearts and leads us to meaningful experiences that our conscious minds cannot even imagine.

This is a story of meaning and values, trust and optimism, gratitude, joy, and good fortune. It happened because I was able to let go and let it happen.

A Story of Kindness

In 1999, one week before I was scheduled to graduate from the Program in Integrative Medicine in Tucson, Arizona, I traveled to Rhinebeck, New York, to the Omega Institute where I took a weeklong workshop on mindfulness-based stress reduction with Jon Kabat-Zinn and Saki Santorelli. While there, I noticed a shop in town that sold musical instruments. I love music (I play the violin) and so I went in to have a look. A few minutes later, I fell in love with a fairly sizeable drum that I thought would be a nice and fun addition to my collection of instruments. Without a thought as to how I would get it home, I bought it and took it back to my room at the institute.

Fast-forward to the following Friday evening, and picture me en route back to Tucson. My plan had been to take the train from Rhinebeck to Pennsylvania Station in New York City where I would grab a taxi to JFK and the plane that would take me home for my graduation the next morning. So far, I had taken the train from Rhinebeck to Penn Station and somehow managed to get my luggage *and* the drum from the train to a street corner outside the station, where I waved frantically as a million taxicabs flew past. Did I mention that it was 5:00 p.m.? And that if I was going to be present for my graduation the next day, I had to catch a 6:45 flight out of JFK?

So there I was, standing on that corner, waving (when I wasn't looking at my watch) and becoming increasingly concerned about missing my plane. A man who looked to be around forty took pity on me and asked if he could help. "You know, you're never going to get a cab," he said. I asked why and he said, "Because it's five o'clock on a Friday and no taxi wants to drive out to JFK. The traffic's awful, so they don't make any money." Then he added, "What you need to do is take the train to the plane. The A line goes right out to JFK." I had no idea what he was talking about and told him so. He said, "Just come with me." He took hold of my drum, walked with me back through the station and down to the subway, where he put two tokens into the turnstile and walked onto the platform with me. When the train arrived, he helped me put my luggage and the drum on and then apologized that he couldn't go with me any farther. I guess he saw the worried expression on my face, because he said, "Don't worry. There will be someone to help you all along the way."

I'd just started worrying about what was next, when a young man and woman asked me where I was going. I explained that I was trying to get to JFK without really knowing the way and that I had just an hour to get there. It didn't look good. The man said, "Don't worry, we'll let you know when it's time to get off." When we pulled into the station, they helped me get my things to the platform and someone getting off the train with me asked if I needed help. He took my drum and got me on the bus that goes directly to the JFK terminal. And so it went. Someone else helped me off the bus and even carried my luggage all the way to the ticket counter. I checked in, boarded the plane, and was at graduation the next morning.

Beyond the miracle of making my flight, I continue to be in awe of the prophetic words of the first man, who'd said, "Don't worry. There will be someone to help you all along the way." That singular, poetic experience is a metaphor for how I became an integrative physician, because all along the way, every time I learned something or gained a new insight, it was because someone else helped me. The experience also resonated with what was happening at the time in integrative medicine, because in those days we were asked to make many great leaps of faith into unknown territory. As we did, life continued to extend its hand in places where we truly needed it.

I think I should mention as a postscript that on the morning of our graduation, my fellow students and I learned that we were each going to be asked to give a small talk. I had nothing prepared, of course. None of us did. So I got up and told the story of my drum and how I got it home. Afterward, everyone said that my few words were the hit of the morning. I was only sorry that the man on the street corner wasn't there to hear it. I think he would have liked it.

PART 3

Your SuperStress Solution

NOW COMES THE FUN PART: transforming ideas and intention into action.

At this point, you know what a stressor is and how myriad stressors bombard us all day long from every direction. You know how subtly, or not so subtly, a stressor lands its punches, and how willingly, or not so willingly, we absorb the blows. You understand how after a while the effects of those blows accumulate until eventually we find ourselves hampered by a bad case of SuperStress.

You even know how SuperStress manifests itself: at first you noticed a backache and thought you must have overdone it when picking up your toddler. At the same time, you experienced a feeling of being overwhelmed and anxious, which you chalked up to an untenable situation at work.

Now you see the big picture, the connection between your mind and your body; now you know that your back pain is most likely *because of* the stress from the untenable situation at work. And that in order to remedy your back pain, you must first pay attention to what is causing your stress and then act on ways to relieve it.

I wrote this book because I want to teach others how to live free of SuperStress. That's what this section of the book is all about. It takes all the information you've learned so far and puts it to work for you, so you can go out into the world and make a better life for yourself.

In this section, you will find two programs that allow you to become active on your own behalf.

The first program is laid out in Chapter 9. This is the Four-Week SuperStress Solution Program that I've previewed throughout this book. It's a comprehensive program designed to attack and reverse the symptoms of SuperStress, and it works well for just about everyone. You'll find simpler programs in Chapter 10, "Superstress Solutions for Your Type," which proposes plans that are more personal in nature, narrower in scope, and address more specific symptoms of SuperStress.

Let's look at each of these programs more closely.

THE FOUR-WEEK SUPERSTRESS SOLUTION PROGRAM

The object of the four-week program is to start you on a trajectory toward wellness and to keep you there long after the twenty-eight days are behind you. It progresses through four weekly themes, each of which builds on the preceding one.

- Week One: Because SuperStressed lives are often out of control, the first week's theme is *Building Calm into Your Life.* You will work toward synchronizing your routines to a saner pace. For example, you will work on getting your sleep patterns and diet under control.
- Week Two. *Detoxifying Mind, Body, and Spirit—and Surroundings,* is about finding tranquility through removing things you find stressful from your life. You'll start to control dietary stimulation and set boundaries with the technologies that tend to overtake your day.
- In Week Three, *Restoring and Rebuilding,* you will begin rebuilding your body's resources by reducing inflammatory agents and boosting your immune system.
- Week Four, *Nurturing Community and the Spirit,* is devoted to relationships—connecting with others and finding your spiritual self.

Each week, you will be encouraged to put a battery of destressing techniques to work: journaling, affirmations, lifestyle habits, physical activity, food, supplements, a mind/body exercise, and a special project. Do you need to use all of these techniques every week? Not if it feels like too much for you. As you know, the last thing I want is for you to get stressed trying to modulate your stress. But keep in mind that the more of these things you *do* put to work, the better you're going to feel. In other words, you'll be more successful if you include physical activity and take advantage of sanctuary moments along with following the food plan than if you follow the food plan alone. Each of my patients has worked the program in a different way, but so far each has been successful.

SUPERSTRESS SOLUTIONS FOR YOUR TYPE

Here I offer a more focused approach to SuperStress. If you choose, for whatever reason, not to do the four-week program, Chapter 10 offers a way to remedy the symptoms of your SuperStress through one of two alternatives. The first of these is comprehensive and is aimed at five different SuperStress Types. People who experience SuperStress tend to fall into one of five types, each of which reflects a mixture of coping styles and the amount of time SuperStress has been untreated. If you took the questionnaires in Chapter 2, you have probably already pinpointed your own type. Are you terribly worn down by your stress, or just a little? Does your coping pattern make you quiet, agitated, angry, scattered, or more controlled? By identifying which type most closely describes your symptoms, you'll quickly find your way to the most effective solution. These types are based on specific behaviors associated with SuperStressed individuals. The second option provides symptom-specific treatments that are helpful as well.

In an ideal world, none of this would be necessary. But we don't live in an ideal world. We all need a bit of help keeping things in perspective from time to time. When you feel yourself losing that perspective, giving in isn't the only choice. In fact, recognizing the problem is a special kind of opportunity: it's an opportunity to begin life anew, wide-awake and fully engaged. Once you start to shed your Super-Stress, your life will become what it was meant to be, full of meaning, value, potential—and peace.

Let's begin. . . .

CHAPTER NINE

The Four-Week SuperStress Solution Program

ALLOW ME TO TAKE you on a brief tour of what awaits you over the next twenty-eight days. As you read earlier, this program progresses through four weekly themes:

WEEK ONE: *Building Calm into Your Life* is designed to relax you and to put you more in control of yourself and your surroundings.

WEEK TWO: *Detoxifying Mind, Body, and Spirit—and Surroundings,* is all about shedding the extraneous issues in your life in preparation for rebuilding a healthier and less-stressed lifestyle.

WEEK THREE: *Restoring and Rebuilding* encourages you now to replace the things that weren't working for you with things healthy and good.

WEEK FOUR: *Nurturing Community and the Spirit* is devoted to relationships. Now that you've restored your balance and are striving to rebuild your life around what truly matters to you, it's time to reach out to others and share yourself with the world.

Although each week is devoted to the central theme, there are common components to the four weeks: journaling, affirmations, lifestyle habits, food, supplements, physical activity, mind/body exercises, and special projects. The following is a brief description of the role each will play in your victory over SuperStress.

JOURNALING

Journaling every day is an excellent tool for self-reflection. It's amazing how much you can learn about yourself simply by observing your thoughts and habits once they're on paper. Also, by recognizing certain patterns, you can avoid those that are not in your best interest.

There are two parts to your journaling exercise: structured dialogue and free-form. *The structured dialogue* is represented by a series of questions that are designed to help you know yourself better. Select one or two of these each day. You'll also see three "essential" questions regarding your daily stress, and these three you are to answer *each day*. The *free-form* journaling is planned dreaming time, which I strongly believe is integral to creativity, gives us spark, and keeps us connected. This is the time to record your dreams from the night before, your thoughts on the day ahead (or just ended), or whatever else comes to mind. You decide what you want to write about and just go to it.

Most of my patients tell me that they find it easiest to journal either in the morning when they awake, or in the evening before bed. Where and when you write in your journal is not as important as it is that you spend twenty or so minutes each day with the TV and radio off, just writing.

AFFIRMATIONS

These daily inspirational mantras are potent tools for change because they reset your subconscious mind to think more positively. Developing a positive mind-set is one of the most powerful life strategies. At a personal level it will transform your life and your health, and renew your joy and passion. Each week you'll find a series of affirmations. Feel free to select any of these or make up your own. (You'll find additional options in Chapter 3.) An affirmation is a declaration that something is true, or that you can turn it into a truth. There are no limits to what you can achieve *if* you keep telling yourself you can.

LIFESTYLE HABITS

It's human nature to do things out of habit, and that's often a good thing, because if we had to make conscious decisions about everything, we'd have no time to rest, dream, imagine, or create. But sometimes we do something mindlessly and *that* becomes habit. Often the habits we fall into are not the healthiest. To reduce or obliterate your Super-Stress, you should be more conscious about your choices so that more healthy emotional and physical habits take root. We all have the opportunity to choose how we live, but in SuperStress people default to survival mode. We're happy just to get through the day, constantly playing catch-up instead of choosing to live a better life. In the next four weeks we'll address the issues of sleep, organization, activity, relaxation, and diet, all of which teach you how to take control over your life.

FOOD: NOURISHING YOUR BODY AND SOUL

In Chapter 4, I explained my philosophy behind eating well. Now we get into the diet. In the appendix, you'll find the SuperStress Solution Diet, which consists of meals plans (twenty-one full-day choices in all) designed to use the stress-fighting foods we discussed earlier. Some of these meal plans are regular or daily menus, and there are also enough choices for a week's worth of the detoxification diet. Here's how the regular diet works over the course of the four-week program.

WEEK ONE: Select what you eat from the regular menus, one for each day.

WEEK TWO: This is the detox week, but you still have choices: you can follow the detox menus, or if you feel that is too stringent, select from the regular menus or try some of each.

WEEKS THREE AND FOUR: Select what you eat each day from the regular menus, or mix and match the meals as you choose.

No matter which menu you choose, do the following every day:

- Try to drink eight glasses of water.
- Have no more than one or two cups of coffee or tea in the morning if you need a pick-me-up (I would prefer that you pick tea, though).
- After lunch, drink a cup of green or herbal tea.
- Drop all processed foods from your diet, including diet soda.
- If you want a snack, have fresh fruit, a handful of nuts, or one ounce of dark chocolate.
- Eat dinner before 7:00 P.M.

Supplements

You'll be using a number of different dietary supplements in the next four weeks. In the Dietary Supplement Health and Education Act (DSHEA) of 1994, Congress defined the term "dietary supplement" as "a product taken by mouth that contains a 'dietary ingredient' intended to supplement the diet." The DSHEA goes on to say: "the 'dietary ingredients' in these products may include: vitamins, minerals, herbs or other botanicals, and amino acids." Dietary supplements may be found in many forms, such as tablets, capsules, gel caps, liquids, or powders. DSHEA places dietary supplements in any form in a special category under the general umbrella of "foods" rather than drugs, and requires that every supplement be labeled as such.

You can find links to general information about dietary and nutritional supplements from the USDA's Food and Nutrition Information Center at http://fnic.nal.usda.gov.

Physical Activity

Here is where you begin to build physical activity into your lifestyle. Physical activity not only relieves stress, it's an exceptional way to diminish unwanted stress hormones. In each of the four weeks, you'll be asked to undertake a walking program and an activity program.

THE WALKING PROGRAM. Your target for the end of the four-week period is 8,000 steps a day. These include your normal "everywhere" steps—to the bakery, the school, strolling with your friends at lunchtime, walking around the office, as well as the steps you take while engaging in the activity program.

You will start with 6,500 steps a day for the first week and increase that by 500 steps a week until you work up to 8,000 by the end. Lest you think you're going to have to count and record steps all day long, take heart! Remember my recommendation of a pedometer? It is a handy gadget that hooks onto your belt and unobtrusively clocks your steps. Put it on first thing in the morning and remove it before bed. A pedometer can be purchased inexpensively at any sporting goods store; other places, such as Wal-Mart, carry them as well. It's actually fun to see how many steps you're taking. If you are short one day, take an extra turn around the block the next day. Or park a little farther from the train station, take five minutes at lunch and walk (this is probably 300 to 500 steps), or climb the stairs instead of taking the elevator. You get the idea. Each week I'll include a grid to record your steps. You may want to copy it into your journal.

THE ACTIVITY PROGRAM. Try to get in twenty to thirty minutes of exercise (other than walking) each day. What you do is up to you, but I made a number of suggestions in Chapter 5 if you run out of ideas. Remember that you can break up your exercise time into five-, ten-, or twenty-minute segments if you need to. Statistics show that you will get the same benefit from exercising in small fragments of time as in one large period, which is why I designed a program for you that includes time-based activities.

Stretching before and after a workout is both relaxing and kind to your muscles. A stretching program is available in Chapter 5.

Drawing on the Mind/Body/Spirit

Each week, you'll use at least two of the exercises in Chapter 3, The Pathways to Peace. These exercises will begin to reset your nervous system to a mode of relaxation and build your resilience. These exercises are as important as any of the others, because the mind and the body are so closely interconnected. To be able to affect the body by drawing on the mind is one of the main principles behind integrative medicine, and one of the essential ways of managing SuperStress.

Your Special Project

Each week you will have one special project to do. The project can be done in a day, a weekend, or whenever you find time and inclination. I've designed them to fit closely into the week's theme, and to be an interesting cap to all that comes before. The main thing is to enjoy yourself with these projects and to come out more relaxed, better organized, less overwhelmed, and feeling better about yourself. Try them. I think you'll be happy you did.

Okay! Are you ready to start the four-week-program?

Great! Let's do it!

WEEK ONE: BUILDING CALM INTO YOUR LIFE

Week One begins an organized strategy designed to move you from a SuperStressed state to a state of serenity. In short: I'm going to teach you how to relax, to bring quiet in the midst of all the craziness that surrounds you (and indeed all of us these days). The theme this week is resetting your inner rhythms by restructuring even the smallest parts of your lifestyle. For example, among the "prescriptions" for the week, you will sleep and wake at a set time in order to get your inner clock back on track. You'll omit unhealthy foods from your diet in an effort to settle down your digestive system, and you'll do mind/body exercises that will nurture the relaxation response.

Start the program by signing the following contract to affirm your commitment to change.

The SuperStress Solution Contract

I, _____, hereby vow that:

    I am committed to improving the quality of my life.

    I acknowledge that I do not have to be perfect.

    Beginning today, I commit to a) doing something, b) thinking something, c) observing something that contributes to my Super-Stress Solution and builds my inner sanctuary.

    I will complete the four-week program.

    Signed _____ Date_____

Journal

Below are your structured questions to answer this week. Recall that they are intended to expand your self-awareness. Answer one a day or, if you prefer, several. Always answer the three essential questions every day.

> *What areas of my life seem out of control?*
> *How do I cope when life gets out of control?*
> *What helps me relax?*
> *What do I love most to do and when was the last time I did this?*
> *What are my goals?*
> *What am I grateful for?*

Answer each of these essential questions *every* day.

> *What stressed me today?*
> *How did I handle the stressor and how did I know I was feeling stressed?*
> *How did I take care of myself after feeling stressed?*

Don't forget to do your daily free-form writing, too. This is your planned dreaming time. Now is the time to write any thoughts that come to your mind about anything. Write in any style you want: it's just you and your journal.

Affirmations

Affirmations work toward developing a positive attitude, even in times when you may not feel so positive. After you have selected your affirmation(s) for the day, don't forget to record them on an index card and place the card in your wallet, tape it on your bathroom mirror, or prop it up on your desk, so you can look at it several times a day. Say the affirmations aloud or silently often.

This week's affirmations:

Abundance is my destiny and I wish this for others as well.
Endless good comes to me in an effortless way.
Every day, I create and appreciate love in my life.
I am an unending reservoir of kindness and peace and release my anger.
I am at peace with myself and with the world.
I am calm and clear-minded.

Lifestyle Habits

This week you're going to focus on what might be an unhealthy habit: how much—or how little—you sleep. Sleeping well is essential to health and carries as much weight as eating well. This week, try to keep to a set sleep schedule. That means going to bed at the same time every night and rising at the same time. The optimal wake/rest cycles are 7:00 A.M. for waking and 11:00 P.M. for retiring. In some writings of Chinese medicine, these hours are associated with staying in harmony with the cycles of nature. If your work schedule makes your suggested wake/rest cycle difficult, do the best that you can to set a routine that works for you.

If you're getting by with five hours of sleep or less, you must evaluate how you can expand those hours, because sleep is a deep-healing time for your body. If you're simply "not a good sleeper," as so many of my patients say they are, go to my "Prescription for Healthy Sleep" and try some of the suggestions (page 99). You'll learn that ambient light disrupts the melatonin cycle that is crucial for deep rest, so it is essential to make sure your sleep area has as little light as possible. It's also a good idea to set up and stick to a bedtime ritual. Patients who have started sleep rituals read inspirational works just before sleeping, journal, or listen to their favorite music or nature sounds. Meditation is another favorite evening event before retiring.

For me, the best unwinding tool is to take a bath with lavender oil soap. I literally wash away the day and turn my attention to being at home. Whatever you choose, the goal is to transition your day from the active (and stressful) awake time to a relaxed and quiet period. In so doing, you're reprogramming your body to understand and respond to downtime as a precursor to sleep.

Relaxing Hot Bath Recipe

Run a very warm bath, and then add a few drops of any of these essential oils:

Lavender	Hops
Marjoram	Valerian
Roman chamomile	

Food: Nourishing Your Body and Soul

This is your first week on the SuperStress Solution Diet. Select a menu each day from the list in the Appendix. Follow this menu plan as closely as you can each day; trying some new recipes will keep things interesting and you may find a few you love. Make a shopping list of the ingredients you'll need and then purchase them at the beginning of the week. Anything to make life simpler.

For this week and every week, do the following:

- Try to drink eight glasses of water each day.
- Have no more than one or two cups of coffee or tea in the morning if you need a pick me-up.
- After lunch, drink a cup of green or herbal tea.
- Drop all processed foods from your diet, including diet soda.
- If you want a snack, have fresh fruit, a handful of nuts, or one ounce of dark chocolate.
- Eat dinner before 7:00 P.M.

Supplements

This week you'll start with a group of supplements that are essential nutritional support for moving out of the SuperStress zone. You won't have to take these indefinitely; as you become less SuperStressed, your need for them will diminish. I have found that, at a minimum, two months and more often, four, are needed to replace the nutrients that are depleted in your body as a result of your SuperStress. Beyond that, it's best to see how you feel. If you still feel a need, you can safely continue to take these supplements indefinitely.

Each of these supplements (and all those you will be taking throughout the four-week plan) can be purchased in either capsule or tablet form unless the prescription calls for a tea or a tincture.

HERE IS YOUR PRESCRIPTION for this week and in fact for every week of the four-week plan. You will be starting here and then building on these as each week continues.

Fish oil. Take 1,000 to 3,000 mg a day. I recommend gel cap form, which comes in 1,000 mg doses. Take one with each meal. This reduces inflammation, which stress can increase.

Magnesium. Take 200 mg a day. This relaxes you but can also create loose stool. If this becomes a problem for you, cut back on the dosage by halving the tablet.

Vitamin B complex, thiamine, pantothenic acid, and folic acid all support metabolism and mood elevation. Note: mg/mcg

B_6. Take 50 to 100 mg a day.

B_{12}. Take 100 to 500 mcg a day under the tongue.

Thiamine. Take 10 mg a day.

Pantothenic acid. Take 10 mg a day.

Folic acid. Take 400 mcg a day (mcg is micrograms, a much smaller dose than milligrams, or mg).

Vitamin D₃. Take 25 mcg to 50 mcg a day (again note that dosage is in micrograms). This enhances the immune system, improves mood regulation, and helps build and maintain healthy bones.

Probiotics. Take 10,000 CFU (colony forming units) a day by capsule. (CFUs are a measurement of the number of organisms in the capsule.) Stress destroys the beneficial flora in the gut. By taking probiotics, you are adding back the flora, which are important for the absorption quality of your intestine.

Physical Activity

Start this week with a goal of walking 6,500 steps per day by the end of the week, and doing at least twenty minutes of exercise daily in addition to the steps. For this week, choose any twenty to thirty minutes of "activity exercises" from Chapter 5, or your own favorites. Remember that you can break down your exercise periods into five-, ten-, or twenty-minute segments and still get the benefits.

Record the number of steps you walk at the end of each day in this chart.

	SUN	MON	TUE	WED	THU	FRI	SAT
Week 1							
Week 2							
Week 3							
Week 4							

Drawing on the Mind/Body/Spirit

This week, start with breathing, which is fundamental to relaxing. If your goal is relaxation, breathing exercises are fundamental. Breathing exercises are the easiest and most portable of all the mind/body exercises because you can practice them anywhere you happen to be. Try any of the breathing exercises in Chapter 3. Mix them up for fun. If you're pressed for time, it's okay to do them in five-minute segments, as many times a day as you feel you need to.

Next, add some meditation. SuperStressed people often can't remember how to relax. They simply can't let go and let life happen. I recognize this situation with patients who tell me that the "sitting still" part of meditation is impossible for them. If that's the case in this first week, you may want to try something else that nurtures inner stillness and yet requires movement, such as tai chi or yoga or playing with a child.

Special Project: Kindness Meditation Practice

This is one of my favorite ways to relax, and, as a bonus, it works wonders in connecting you to the world.

Kindness Meditation Practice

Sit in a comfortable chair with your body relaxed and your mind at rest. Try to think only of where you are right now. Begin reciting the following phrases. You're wishing yourself well because you must love yourself first if you are ever to love others.

> *May I be filled with lovingkindness.*
> *May I be well.*
> *May I be peaceful and at ease.*
> *May I be happy.*

Say these phrases to yourself three times. It helps to visualize an image of yourself as you are saying them. Imagine that this image of yourself is sending you love and well wishes. When you feel ready, let this image fade and imagine someone living or dead who has truly cared for you. Say the phrases above three times, sending love to your person as you say them: *May he/she be filled with loving-*

kindness. May he/she be well. . . . As you do this, imagine that you are receiving love in return. Let this image fade and then picture someone with whom you have had great difficulty. Send them the same warmth and love that you just sent the person who loves you. Now imagine that person returning love and wishing you well. Repeat the phrase three times. When you are ready, let this image fade and include anyone in your immediate surroundings in your wishes. Repeat the phrases wishing them well, and as you do send them love and receive their well wishes. Next, include your friends and coworkers. Then include your neighbors. In time, wish this lovingkindness to people in your city, your state, your country, and your planet. Within a fifteen-minute period, you will have wished lovingkindness to all the world. As you silently practice this meditation, allow yourself to enjoy the sensation of an immediate connection with everyone you encounter in your thoughts. This awareness gives you the opportunity to appreciate all the people directly and indirectly connected to you. At the end, you will feel a profound and expansive sense of goodness and grace toward humanity, our planet, and beyond. Guaranteed.

WEEK TWO: DETOXIFYING MIND, BODY, AND SPIRIT—AND SURROUNDINGS

Week Two is all about cleaning out the elements in your life that are obstacles to tranquility of the mind, body, and spirit. Because this is your detoxification week, you're going to be leaving behind things that don't serve you well. This week you will begin to take short breaks throughout the day so that even if you are not aware of your stress, you will still moderate it by stopping what you're doing and listening to your inner thoughts. Week Two also introduces the detoxification diet, designed to help reduce toxins in your body while simultaneously providing sufficient nourishment. For this week I also offer you a variety of alternative or indigenous healing modalities that will encourage your wound-up nervous system to unwind and let go.

Journaling

Here are some new questions to ask yourself. Select one or more of these to answer daily.

What lifted my spirits today?
What did I do to support myself?
What am I grateful for?
What insight did I gain from today?
What did I do to relax?

Answer each of these essential questions *every* day.

What stressed me today?
*How did I handle the stressor and how did I know I was feeling
   stressed?*
How did I take care of myself after feeling stressed?

Don't forget to enjoy your daily free-form writing, too.

Affirmations

Here are some new affirmations to record in your journal and to put on your mirror, in your wallet, or on your desk at work. Saying them to yourself or aloud will reinforce the affirmation.

I have the power to take charge of my life.
I have unlimited choices that bring me serenity with every step.
Peace is within me and fills my heart with every breath.
There is a divine plan for me and I am open to watching it unfold.
I feel the stillness within myself.
I give myself permission to realize my dreams.
I have a lot to give, and I enjoy giving.

Lifestyle Habits

As part of your detoxification week, you need to begin to curb your exposure to and absorption of the negative energy and negative thoughts that come at all of us through the local, national, and world news. Toward this end:

- Watch the evening news for no more than thirty minutes.
- Start limiting your PDA and cell phone use by shutting both off during meals and creating at least one twenty-minute PDA- and phone-free hiatus in your day, every day!
- As much as possible, stay away from people who don't bring you joy. To my mind, negative people can do as much damage to us as spending a week listening to nothing but bad news from around the world.

Start to build points of stillness into each day. This week schedule two sacrosanct stop-everything-you're-doing ten-minute breaks at work, in which you do one of the following.

- Do a simple breath exercise (see Chapter 3) and blow those toxins out of your system.
- Prepare a cup of tea and drink it while visualizing a beautiful place where you feel at peace.
- Get out of the office to walk around the block, inhaling the "good" air and exhaling the "bad."
- Go off by yourself and listen to some soothing music, or better still, take a walk and listen to the sounds of nature.

Food: Nourishing Your Body and Soul

Hundreds of scientific studies tell us that stress leads to overeating and most of that is unhealthy food. Consequently, many of us have bodies that are overloaded with chemicals that are better off eliminated. This week I have put together a seven-day detoxification diet that offers the choice of a primarily liquid diet or a simplified macrobiotic version. Try one or the other or a few days of each. If the detox diet feels too stringent or if you have any reason not to make use of it, repeat the first week of the regular menus, but scale down the portions. The less you eat, the less work for your liver.

For this week and every week on the diet, do the following:

- Try to drink eight glasses of water each day.
- Have no more than one or two cups of coffee or tea in the morning if you need a pick-me-up.
- After lunch, drink a cup of green or herbal tea.
- Drop all processed foods from your diet, including diet soda.
- If you want a snack, have fresh fruit, a handful of nuts, or one ounce of dark chocolate.
- Eat dinner before 7:00 P.M.

Supplements

The liver is the body's waste management center. Day in and day out it modifies all the nutrients and chemicals in the bloodstream. In this, your detox week, I am adding four new supplements, each with the intent of reinforcing your liver's ability to function during any overwork it might entail. You can also flush toxins from your body by drinking a lot of water. Try for eight glasses a day in addition to any other liquid you might be consuming.

Continue the first week's supplements, but this week add the four I itemize below, which are specifically supportive of your liver. Even if you are not on the detoxification diet, you'll give your liver a boost by using these supplements, which come in either tablet or capsule form.

> *Milk thistle* (Silybum marianum). Take 240 mg three times a day.
> *Turmeric* (Curcuma longa). Take 1000 mg four times a day.
> *Alpha lipoic acid.* Take 600 mg a day.
> CoQ_{10}. Take 100 mg a day.

Physical Activity

If you're on the detox diet, you may not want to engage in too much physical activity beyond your walking program this week, but there are still many things you can do. On or off the detox diet, continue your walking. This week, try to reach 7,000 steps a day by the end of the week. (You can chart your progress on the walking grid on page 190.) If you're not on the detox diet, do the walking program and set aside twenty to thirty minutes each day for one of the exercises listed in Chapter 5. Or try an aerobic activity, such as a bicycle ride, a step class, or a Pilates class. Doing so will get you out of the house and engaged with others as you increase your lung capacity and build a stronger heart. A triple winner!

Drawing on the Mind/Body/Spirit

It's all about calmness and serenity. Begin to build "still points" at least twice a day by sitting in a quiet place, closing your eyes, and spending at least ten minutes on one or more of the following exercises to clear your mind and bring it to a more tranquil place. Try any of these meditations once a day or twice if you're lucky enough to have the time.

- Visualization: imagine yourself in a beautiful place where you feel at peace.
- Object-focused meditation: train your full concentration on a pleasing object, tuning out all other thoughts.
- Sound meditation: train your full concentration on a pleasing sound, like the crash of waves or the flow of a fountain.
- Breath meditation: sit in meditation position and choose a positive word like *peace* or *love* or *calm* to concentrate on with each inhalation and another to say when exhaling.

Special Project: Sleep Like a Baby

As you are detoxifying your body, you are also going to detox your environment. Last week you spent time on changing your sleep habits. This week's project is to transform your sleeping space into an arena of Zenlike serenity. The bedroom is a vital place of restoration and peace. If yours is not as tranquil as you'd like, take some time and put it in order. Do you bring work into your sleeping space? Not this week, you don't. This is a week for removing from your sleeping area anything that's too bright, loud, or distracting. Are there things that you don't like to look at that you've been meaning to remove—such as a photograph of an old boyfriend? How about that tattered bathrobe hanging on the hook across from the bed? Banish them from your sight. Put the detractors in a closet. Give them to a friend. Just get rid of them. And then snuggle in for the best night's sleep you've had in years.

More Than Just Pretty to Look At . . .

It is well known that plants can contribute to cleaning and detoxifying the air. In a NASA study investigating plants that have this ability, five were noted to be the most effective. You may want to add them to your home:

Mass cane (*Dracaena massangeana*)

Pot mum (*Chrysanthemum morifolium*)

Gerbera daisy (*Gerbera jamesonii*)

Warneckii (*Dracaena deremensis* 'Warneckii')

Ficus (*Ficus benjamina*)

WEEK THREE: RESTORING AND REBUILDING

Disorganization is a common by-product (as well as a promoter) of SuperStress. Research has shown that we secrete cortisol when we're surrounded by disarray. So this week you will be focusing on reclaiming control in your environment as well as other critical areas of your life. In Week Two, you eliminated distracting mind clutter in the bedroom, making it more peaceful. This week you're extending that process to include all of your surroundings. Once the confusion and disorder is eliminated, you can start to rebuild your environment to reflect and reinforce a simpler life.

Journal

Here are some new questions to try to answer through your journaling this week.

What is cluttering my life?
Why have I not changed it?
What areas of my life seem out of control?
What has been most meaningful to me over the past two weeks?
What have I learned that will be helpful to me going forward?

Answer each of these essential questions *every* day.

What stressed me today?
How did I recognize I was stressed?
How did I take care of myself after feeling stresssed?

Because we're thinking now of rebuilding your life, you may want to work on your goals instead of free-form journaling. Note areas of your life that seem out of control. Use the "Transitions and Goals" template diagram below to make a plan to repair them. Keep your goals small and realistic so they don't overwhelm you, and accomplish at least three of them by the week's end. You'll be surprised how much of a difference small accomplishments make when it comes to restoring your feelings of control. Notice that I suggest breaking your goals into increments of short-term (one day), near future (this week), distant future (this month), and long-term (this year) time frames. Breaking your goals down this way will help you figure out how to make changes and plan for ways to turn your goals into realities.

Transitions and Goals

Changes to Make in:	One Day	This Week	This Month	This Year
Environment				
Workplace				

Relationships

_____

_____

_____

_____

Health and Habits

_____

_____

_____

Dreams and Creativity

_____

_____

Affirmations

Remember to log a new affirmation into your journal this week, and to post or keep your choice somewhere you'll see it regularly (on your desk, on a mirror, in your wallet). Here are some new affirmations you might find inspiring.

> *I can manage my time.*
> *I can sit quietly without fidgeting or ruminating.*
> *I cast difficult burdens up to the greater good and see new opportunities in unusual situations.*
> *I draw strength from the people I love, and I give it back.*
> *I have all the tools I need to master my concerns.*
> *I deserve peace and fulfillment.*
> *I deserve to devote time to my personal life.*

Lifestyle Habits

Now is the time to get rid of unnecessary things, simplify our lives, and gain clarity about what's really important to us, and why we do the things we do. For people with SuperStress who feel as if they never have enough time—and that includes just about all of them—it's essential to understand where that time goes. Why do we do what we do? Sometimes the answer is: just because we feel like it. That's perfectly reasonable, as long as you understand that spending time on a particular undertaking is your choice.

To help you see that you do have choices about how you spend your time, take a clean sheet of paper and jot down the things you have on tap for every day this week—work, laundry, picking up the kids, lunch with a friend, shopping, gym, and so forth. As you go through each day, add the things you do that you have not planned, such as spending a half hour on the telephone with someone you hardly know or stopping in a bookstore to browse just because you pass it on the way to the supermarket. (These are things that might take time away from your priorities but that might also be pressure valves during the day, and as such—helpful!) Then, at the end of the day, assign a priority level to each task you performed and the unexpected things you did.

- Essential
- Essential but can be delegated
- Not essential but done because of fear of disapproval or a sense of obligation
- Not essential but carried out anyway (list why, including fun, curiosity, seemed like a good idea at the time, just felt like it . . .)

This should give you a fairly good idea of how you're spending your time, and why. It will also help you arrange your priorities in the future.

Food: Nourishing Your Body and Soul

In Week Three you will again select daily eating plans from the regular menus. Because this is the "restore and rebuild" week, it's time to renew your relationship with yourself. To this end, select one day this week where you plan a special meal for just you alone. Set the table with flowers and your best china. Turn on some relaxing music. Dim the lights or put candles on the table. Then, spend at least one hour eating and paying attention to each bite you take, chewing slowly and deliberately and noticing the texture and taste of the food. As you eat, take your time and pay attention to your thoughts and to every bite you take. Try to remember this meal in the future when you think it's necessary to gulp down your meals to get to the next task at hand.

For this week and every week, do the following:

- Try to drink at least eight glasses of water each day.
- Have no more than one or two cups of coffee or tea in the morning if you need a pick-me up.
- After lunch, drink a cup of green or herbal tea.
- Drop all processed foods from your diet, including diet soda.
- If you want a snack, have fresh fruit, a handful of nuts, or one ounce of dark chocolate.
- Eat dinner before 7:00 P.M.

Supplements

This third week brings a few more changes to your supplement intake.

Here is your prescription for the week:

Continue the first week's supplements. Since you are no longer on the detox diet, you can stop taking the milk thistle, turmeric, alpha lipoic acid, and the CoQ_{10}.

For the next two weeks, add the following supplements:

Astragalus: Take 4 to 7 grams a day in capsule form.

Astragalus membranaceus is an herb that has been used in Chinese medicine for hundreds of years. My grandfather used it in our family soup recipe—the one that I used to deliver by hand to our neighbors when I was a little girl. *Astragalus* has immune-boosting properties; there are even a few small studies indicating that it is useful in reducing the risk of the common cold. In this, our rebuilding week, note that *Astragalus* is also useful for rebuilding two areas of the body that are highly vulnerable to the stress response hormones: the immune system and the intestines.

Host Defense: Take 2 capsules a day. Host Defense is a blend of medicinal mushrooms. It is manufactured by Fungi Perfecti, LLC, a dietary supplement company. (Products are available at www.fungi.com.) This product is a combination of Reishi, Maitake, *Cordyceps,* shiitake, and Zhu Ling mushrooms. Each kind of mushroom has been shown to have immunity-enhancement properties in its own right; the blend here is particularly healing. There are other medicinal mushroom products—for instance, pure preparations of Maitake or Reishi mushrooms—that you can substitute as your choice for Host Defense if you like.

The length of time you take *Astragalus* and Host Defense will depend on how worn down your immune system is. If you are getting sick for the first time or feeling vulnerable to illness as a result of fatigue, then two weeks is an adequate period. If you have been getting viral illness after viral illness, my suggestion would be to take both these supplements for at least two to three months—as long as you let your health care provider know you are doing this. That's because this is an immunity tonic, and if you're taking something for a prolonged period and have any immune-related problems, your physician should know about it.

Physical Activity

Your walking program should reach 7,500 steps per day this week. For your other activity, try doing the full-body workout (page 115) three days. Commit the other four days to taking the stairs instead of the elevator for the entire day. If by some chance you never have a need to take the stairs, find a building that has them and walk up and down for a half hour each day. Not only will this count toward your total steps, but you'll get a full aerobic benefit as well.

Drawing on the Mind/Body/Spirit

Try something different this week. Go to Chapter 3 and read down the list of mind/body exercises. Experiment with a different one each day. Perhaps try a tai chi lesson or have a massage. Or go for the Kirtan Kriya meditation where you chant for five or ten minutes. Progressive muscle relaxation exercise might be fun, too. Experiment. Enjoy.

Project: Organize for a Stress-Free Life

Take one half day this week and dedicate it to a cleaning or organizing project you've been wanting to do, *as long as in the end you have less clutter than you started with*. Remember, this is the week for rebuilding. Here are some suggestions for tasks that will make you feel great when you have completed them: clean your closets, straighten up your basement, or organize your photos, recipes, and household paperwork. When you're done, celebrate with a smoothie of your choice! (See Appendix.)

WEEK FOUR: NURTURING COMMUNITY AND THE SPIRIT

Disconnection from loved ones, the world, and your creativity is both a symptom and a cause of SuperStress. In this final week, you'll concentrate on reestablishing the linkages that make us feel like active participants in our own lives. This is a time to ask the bigger questions: *What am I living for? Is this where I want to be? What really matters? Am I making a difference?* It's a time to do something kind for someone this week—just because. Make a lunch date with a friend or your spouse, or most important, with the loved ones you adore but never seem to have time for because you know *they will always be there*. But will they? Who knows? Don't wait a second longer. Call these people today and make that important date. This week, you'll also be concerned with strangers. Perform random acts of kindness for people whom you have never met. If you think that connecting with a loved one makes you feel good—and it surely does—wait until you see how amazing you feel after doing an unexpected kindness for a stranger.

Journal

You will be asked in the project section of this week to do some random acts of kindness. As you do, record what they were and how you felt afterward. On days six and seven of this week, write how you feel after having completed this program.

Answer some of the following questions earlier in the week.

Where do I see myself in a year?
Where do I see myself in three years?
*When was the last time I told a loved one how much he or she means
    to me?*

Now that you're into week four, I'm going to assume your stress has diminished significantly, so instead of your daily writings about your stress, this week record for each day:

A *moment of meaning*
A *moment of gratefulness*
A *moment of giving*

Remember that these moments can be small, and that small changes add up to big ones.

Affirmations

You've worked hard these past weeks and now instead of surviving, you're thriving! After all this time on the program, I would hope that these affirmations ring true.

I am worthy of happiness.
I can achieve the peace I desire.
I can attract the life and love I want.
I can feel the stillness within myself.
I can honestly appraise my life and make positive changes.

Lifestyle Habits

This week, you'll focus on habits that affect your health. Have you checked in with your primary care doctor in the last year? If not, I suggest you make an appointment for a complete physical examination. While you are at it, you may want to make a few more appointments for yourself. How about making a call a day to schedule each of these, if you need to:

- Monday: Make an appointment for a pap smear if you are a woman over eighteen or a prostate screening if you are a man over forty.
- Tuesday: Make an appointment for a mammogram screening if you are female and over forty.
- Wednesday: Make an appointment for a colonoscopy if you are older than fifty and have not had one yet.
- Thursday: Consider getting a bone density test if you are female, over fifty, and have not had one, or if it has been five years since your last scan.
- Friday: Check on your need to update your vaccinations.

Feels good, doesn't it?

Food: Nourishing Your Body and Soul

This week, select your diet for the day from the regular menus. Make your last evening this week a celebratory one. Select the festive meal menu and invite some family or friends to join you. Celebrate your togetherness and join hands before dinner in gratitude for one another.

For this week and every week on the diet, do the following:

- Try to drink eight glasses of water each day.
- Have no more than one or two cups of coffee or tea in the morning if you need a pick-me-up.
- After lunch, drink a cup of green or herbal tea.
- Drop all processed foods from your diet, including diet soda.
- If you want a snack, have fresh fruit, a handful of nuts, or one ounce of dark chocolate.
- Eat dinner before 7:00 P.M.

Supplements

You are in your last week, but you can feel free to continue any of these supplements for as long as you think they're helpful.

Here is your prescription for the week:

Repeat your supplement program from week three, continuing with the *Astragalus* (4 to 7 grams a day) and the Host Defense (2 capsules a day).

Physical Activity

This week you are going to reach your goal of 8,000 steps a day! You want to do more? *GO FOR IT!* Wearing your pedometer will help you rack up those steps, especially if you opt for climbing the stairs to your office or taking that long walk at lunch. In addition, try to fit in thirty minutes of exercise daily this week. Just remember that you have choices for how and when to exercise: Six five-minute stints, three ten-minute stints. Thirty minutes, no matter how you slice it!

Because this is a week devoted to connection, I suggest that one of your exercises this week be dancing. Take along a friend or loved one and find a place where you can hit the dance floor and let loose. (Or, at a minimum, take one of your walks with a friend.) Also, you might take classes at a gym and enjoy exercising in the company of others. If you're not a member of a gym, ask a friend if you can be a guest. Some gyms will offer a free one-day trial to prospective members, so that's another way to find people to exercise with.

Because this week is also devoted to spirituality, take a walk in the park. Don't listen to music. Listen to the sounds of nature. Go to the beach alone and hear the crashing of the waves. Nature belongs to all of us. It's free. And it's beautiful. And it will lift your spirits.

Drawing on the Mind/Body/Spirit

This week, do your mind/body exercises with someone you love on as many days as you can. Sing together. Drum together. In many cultures, drumming is a community effort. Take a yoga class with your siblings or your children. Even better, play *with* some children: play hopscotch with the neighbors' daughter, or jump on a trampoline with your son, or tumble with your pets. Have a great time! It's refreshing for the mind and the soul.

You might also want to teach Kritan Kriya (see Chapter 3) to a group of your friends. Get a massage. Get two! Nothing relaxes like the assured touch of a professional masseuse. If you have a partner, get massages together; even though it's quiet time, you'll still be interacting with another person.

SPECIAL PROJECT: DOING WELL BY DOING GOOD

Week Four's project reflects on your spirituality. In Chapter 8, the last "tools" chapter, you connected spirituality to values, meaning, and, in some cases, prayer. So it seems appropriate that you should end your four-week program, which has done you so much good, by giving back to others. And when you do, you will personally gain, because the interaction is in its own way a true SuperStress remedy.

This week, do the following random acts of kindness for seven days. Perform one a day, or seven in one day. The more you do, the better you'll feel, and the stronger your connection to yourself and those who matter most to you. I'm certain you can conjure up many acts of kindness of your own. Be observant as you go through your day and when opportunity strikes, seize the opportunity to do some good. It will pay you back many times over.

Here are some ideas, but I believe that once you get started, you'll think of many more on your own.

- Send a donation to your favorite charity.
- Write a real, old-fashioned longhand letter to someone just to catch up.
- Go out of your way to say hello to or help a neighbor.
- Read a story to your child or someone else's.
- Stand back and hold open a door for someone you would normally rush by.
- Smile at a stranger.
- Offer to help someone you don't know because they look as if they could use your assistance.

Assessing Your Week

After your four weeks of attending to your physical, emotional, and spiritual needs, it's a great time to retake the four self-diagnostic questionnaires (pages 42 to 50) to see how your life has changed. Do it now, and then again in one month, and again in a year to see whether you need a refresher course on achieving serenity. If you do, you can repeat the entire program, if you wish, or even just your favorite week.

CHAPTER TEN

SuperStress Solutions for Your Type

IF YOU DON'T WANT TO PARTAKE of the four-week plan I've just outlined—and I recognize that one plan can never fit everyone's needs—you can still reap some of its stress-reduction benefits by dipping into this simplified version, a toolbox of stand-alone solutions for your SuperStress type and also a list of remedies for your specific symptoms.

You will have already identified your SuperStress Type if you have answered the questions in the questionnaires in Chapter 2. If you have not yet filled out the questionnaires, go back and do so now. After you learn which type you are, put to use the type-specific tools that will best help with your issues. If you can't easily see yourself in any of these types, you might instead be able to identify a single physical or emotional symptom that's bothering you most. If that's the case, skip ahead to page 220 where I will itemize SuperStress Tools to use in defense against the most common specific symptoms. First, though, let's look at the five SuperStress types.

TYPE I: BURNED OUT, EXHAUSTED, NUMB, DEPRESSED

Profile: Do you experience extreme fatigue when you awaken in the morning and then throughout the day? Perhaps you're like the soccer mom with five young children who feels she's fighting a losing battle trying to keep up with their sports schedules, French lessons, dental appointments, and homework. Or the lawyer who sits through a partners' meeting trying to look interested, while struggling to keep his thoughts from drifting. If instead of enjoying your family, all you long for is the end of the day and a few minutes to yourself, or if either of these earlier descriptions sounds familiar, you can consider yourself a categorical Type I. You've reached the point where stress has been present for so long that you can no longer mount a reaction to any stressors. But all is not lost. You will definitely find help for your symptoms in the prescriptions below.

Diet: Eating right will go a long way toward moderating the effects of the continual surge of stress hormones that cascade through the bodies of people with Type I SuperStress. (This holds true for the other four types as well.) That's because one of the most dangerous physical consequences of SuperStress is inflammation, and it has been proven that certain foods can help the body defend against this unwelcome byproduct. Type Is generally do well on a diet that's strongly vegetarian, though fish is permitted. Steamed dark greens appear to be particularly helpful. I suggest that those of you who feel burned out or as if you're running on empty should start your day with a high-antioxidant, whey-based breakfast shake with 2 teaspoons of coconut oil, 1 tablespoon of wheat germ, and 2 teaspoons of nut butter. If you want something more substantial, try warm cereal with a tablespoon of wheat germ and a tablespoon of ground flaxseed. You can design your own meal plan or select from those I've included in the appendix. It's up to you. Oh, and here's some good news: you get to have one ounce of dark chocolate every day if you want it—without guilt. Dark chocolate is a wonderful tool, not only for quick energy, but for beating back inflammation, too. Eat it in bar form or drink it as hot chocolate. Just don't go overboard.

I'm a great proponent of tea. Three to five cups of green tea will help to soothe you throughout the day and will also keep you focused. So why not take a few minutes for yourself and savor both the tea and the time for yourself as you sip it? Then, at the end of the day, put your feet up, relax, and enjoy your last cup of green tea. That's what I do, whenever I get the chance.

Supplements: Below I've suggested what may at first appear to be a large number of supplements, but understand that you can take as many or as few of them as you want, and for as long a period as suits your needs. There is no problem taking any of these supplements at the same time. Or beginning with a few and adding more as you go along.

All supplements can be found in either tablet or capsule form, unless otherwise specified, such as those to be used in teas or tinctures (oil).

- For general anti-inflammatory support, take 1 g of omega-3 fatty acid fish oil and 1 g of turmeric a day.
- For increased energy support, try low-dose *Rhodiola* or low-dose Siberian ginseng. *Rhodiola* and Siberian ginseng are herbs that give increased energy and stamina, and elevate mood. A starting dose for Rhodiola is 100 to 300 mg daily and Siberian ginseng 1 to 2 g a day.
- For immune stabilization, take *Astragalus,* 10 to 20 grams a day *and* Reishi mushrooms in capsules of 1 to 1.5 grams a day. These can be taken separately or together.
- For a more solid, settled, and calm sleep at night, take 1 mg of melatonin and/or 100 mg of L-theanine. These should be taken an hour before going to bed.
- For mild depression, take 300 mg Saint-John's-wort three times a day.
- Every morning, take the following vitamins for overall stress support:
  - Vitamin B_{12}, 1,000 mcg under the tongue
  - Folic acid A, 800 mcg
  - Biotin, 500 to 1,000 mcg
- For your relaxing evening cup of tea, boil some hot water and add 10 to 15 drops of tincture of either valerian, hops, kava, or passion flower.

Exercise: Here's a great way to energize yourself. Strap on your pedometer and try to walk at least 6,000 steps a day. In addition, schedule an hour of yoga or a Pilates class at least once a week. Or, for more fun, try an energizing dance or aerobics class for forty-five minutes. Sometimes just being in a group of people is all that it takes to lift your spirits, and who knows? You might just make a new friend or two to bring new interests into your life.

Special Strategies: If you're a Type I, even though you feel burned out, you will benefit greatly from relaxation exercises. For you, both energy and calmness can be derived from a good massage. My favorite has always been a hot stone or Thai massage, but any type will do. (Just make sure your masseuse is licensed.) Those of you who are feeling a bit depressed might want to engage in acupuncture or Reiki therapy. If you have access to a sauna, I highly recommend spending time in it at least once a week.

TYPE II: AGITATED, OVERWHELMED BY LIFE

Profile: Irritated and irritatible to distraction? Does a simple to-do list of four items or fewer seem daunting? Do you find yourself reading the same paragraph over and over and feeling increasingly frustrated that you just don't get it? If these definitions describe you, you're certainly in good company these days. While you may not be exactly like, say, the investment banker who's trying to support her family while simultaneously keeping her clients happy in a spiraling-out-of-control economic market, you might well share her mind-set. If you have days when your agitation is so great that you're distracted by your own restlessness, if you dream of the days when sleep came easily to you, well then you, dear reader, are a typical Type II. The good news is: you can plan on turning those dreams into reality, because I have just the solution for you.

Diet: To moderate the undesirable effects of a system overtaxed by stress hormones, I suggest you consume a diet that works against inflammation. That is a basically Mediterranean-style diet with an emphasis on simple protein (mostly fish), whole grains, fruits, vegetables, and olive oil. (You can find these foods described in more detail in Chapter 4.) Start the day with a high-antioxidant, whey-based shake with 2 tablespoons of ground flaxseed and 1 tablespoon of wheat germ, or hot cereal with a tablespoon each of ground flaxseed and wheat germ, plus ½ cup of fresh fruit.

Because your symptoms include being overwhelmed and agitated, calm is the byword. I associate calm with tea, and I recommend that you indulge in five cups of green tea or herbal tea a day, if only for the calming effect. But don't just wolf it down. The object of drinking tea, aside from its antioxidant properties, is that it requires that you take out a few minutes both to brew it and to sip it—minutes that will distract you from your other tasks and help reset your inner time clock. Space out the five cups of tea—either green tea or chamomile tea, sweetened with honey if you choose—over the course of the day and evening. As you indulge in your tea, put your work aside and do nothing more than think about the fact that you are doing something good for yourself. Somewhere during the day, you should also enjoy one ounce of dark chocolate, which has been increasingly shown to be a healthy indulgence. Oh, and did I mention the word *delicious*?

Supplements:
- For general anti-inflammatory support, start with omega-3 fatty acid fish oil, 2 grams a day.
- For calming, try the amino acid 5 hydroxytryptophan (5-HTP)— 100 mg twice a day. (Note: Avoid if taking an antidepressant.)
- To support sleep, before bed take 1 mg of melatonin, 100 mg of L-theanine, and a cup of chamomile tea with honey.
- For general antioxidant support, take daily:
    - A multivitamin, plus
    - Vitamin B_{12}, 1000 mcg under the tongue
    - Folic acid A , 800 mcg
    - Biotin, 500 to 1,000 mcg

Exercise: To help you calm down and regroup, I suggest at least twenty minutes a day of brisk walking or jogging (broken up into five- or ten-minute segments if you need to) or a half hour of swimming, which will also do the trick. For fun—and who among us doesn't need a little fun these days?—you may want to engage in a group game such as basketball or tennis every so often. The exercise is great for what ails you and the companionship is a wonderful way to remind you of what's important in life.

Special Strategies: Acupuncture, massage, or an hour of yoga or tai chi will go a long way toward calming you down. Meditation is great, too. It's free, and requires nothing more than time, so I suggest you look at Chapter 3 and select one of the four types of meditation included there. It may take you awhile to get the hang of it. Even in the beginning, though, there is nothing but good that can come from engaging in some form of meditation.

TYPE III: EMOTIONALLY SENSITIVE

Profile: Remember what it was like to be a senior in high school? Stressed over college applications, hating your body, believing the whole world thought you were a nerd? I remember. And I remember that it wasn't always fun. But I am often reminded of it by so many of my patients, who report experiencing the same feelings, if in different circumstances. Say, for instance, a marketing executive's boss tells her that her report needs more work. Right away, she interprets those words to mean: "My boss hates me. He thinks I'm worthless." No, I'll remind her. Your boss just didn't like your *report*. Or I find myself saying to an insecure medical student, "Perhaps your girlfriend really was busy on Friday night." Do they believe me? Of course not. These reactions are common in a Type III, so it doesn't surprise me when their reaction to SuperStress is feeling emotionally vulnerable or especially sensitive to criticism. The Type III has lost a sense of humor and tends to be weepy or melancholy. If you recognize yourself in this type, I'm guessing that every little stressor finds its way directly to your stomach. Every knock to your self-esteem creates an emotional turmoil that hits your digestion. When that happens, your stomach or intestinal functions exhibit signs of strain, causing a gassy, bloated feeling that's accompanied by stomach cramps, loose stools, or constipation. All typical symptoms of irritable bowel syndrome, or IBS. These suggestions will help you get out of that undesirable state:

Diet: If you're a Type III, you will do well to stay with a simple Mediterranean type diet (small amounts of low-fat animal protein and seafood and lots of greens and ripe fruits), because these foods work to correct a bloated belly. Just remember not to eat too fast, and don't talk while chewing your food. (Really. Swallowing air is one sure way to bloat the belly.) Increase your turkey consumption because the tryptophan in turkey is calming. Some people believe that tryptophan is the reason why we want to go to sleep right after a lovely Thanksgiving dinner, but I'm not sure that's anything more than just a rumor. This doesn't hold true for chicken, however. Note that increasing chicken consumption is not the same thing as eating turkey, because chicken, especially dark meat, is more inflammatory. It contains a lot of arachidonic acid, a molecule that increases inflammation. Fennel tea reduces bloating, so try to have it at least once or twice daily. Hawthorn berry tea is a mild diuretic so it is helpful, too. Also eat vegetables such as steamed kale, dandelion greens, and Swiss chard.

Supplements:
- For anti-inflammatory support and to stabilize moodiness, take omega-3 fatty acid fish oil, 1 g a day.
- For calming purposes, take 200 mg magnesium glycinate twice a day.
- For general vitamin support, take daily:
  - Vitamin B_{12}, 1,000 mcg under the tongue
  - Biotin, 500 to 1,000 mcg
  - Vitamin B_6, 25 to 50 mg
  - Vitamin C, 500 to 1,000 mg
  - Vitamin D_3, 25 to 50 mcg

Exercise: Start with a simple walking routine at a comfortable speed for twenty minutes a day. The object is to pace your nervous system, so the emphasis is on walking every day, rather than on how far or how fast you go. If you want to add more exercise, go to Chapter 5 and select anything that you feel would be enjoyable. Again, try to do something every day even if only for a short period. Exercise is great for raising your self-esteem, and it keeps your digestion moving along, too. Both are desirable end products for the person with Type III Super-Stress.

Special Strategies: For the sensitive person, positive affirmations seem to work wonders. It's never too soon to start reminding yourself of all your strengths. Write them down and take a good long look at all the things you are proud of. Next, create a script for a tape of affirmations, in which you read them over a background of your favorite music. Play this tape on a daily basis while doing a progressive relaxation exercise. You can create new scripts as you go along and as you begin to feel better about yourself. A second tape might reflect your own vision of serenity, and this you can play in the evening for relaxation before bedtime.

TYPE IV: DRIVEN, CONTROLLING

Profile: If you're a Type IV person, you are first-rate at setting a goal and going full steam ahead until you reach it. Here's the bad news: Type IVs are generally work-obsessed, so after a while, goal achievement, overattention to detail, and a tendency toward micromanagement become the only ways they can handle situations that feel out of control. One of the first patients whom I defined as truly SuperStressed was a workaholic magazine editor in chief who wanted to be in charge of every situation and employee she came into contact with. And she *knew* she was doing it. But she continued anyway. She felt Super-Stressed because she was falling increasingly behind at work. Also, she explained to me, she couldn't understand why her coworkers would rather go home at the end of the day than have a social drink with her. Type IV behavior ultimately crowds out other, healthier parts of life, such as family and friends. Type IVs put most social activities and key relationships on the back burner. If you're one who approaches your life in this manner, I'm willing to bet you have symptoms that reflect this tension, such as constipation, neck pain, back pain, and stomach problems.

Diet: If you're a Type IV, the best eating plan for you is based on the Mediterranean-style eating plan. Special protein foods that are helpful for you are turkey (full of tryptophan, which possibly enhances serotonin, which in turn enhances calmness), cold-water fish, and legumes, particularly black beans. Other foods that serve as replenishing starches are grains like millet, rice, and quinoa. Root crops, such as beets and sweet potatoes, are beneficial because they are good sources of fiber. Other fiber sources that coat the stomach with a natural protective lubricant are flaxseed (ground), fenugreek, and psyllium. Minimize raw foods and keep your diet simple, without elaborate sauces.

Supplements: Because Type IV patients so often have associated bowel problems, I always start them on a probiotic. A probiotic is a supplement that contains acidophilus and lactobacillus species, both of which provide healthy digestive organisms to the GI tract.

- Take approximately 6 million to 10 million colony-forming units (CFU) of a probiotic daily (on an empty stomach).
- For anti-inflammatory support, take omega-3 fatty acid fish oil, 1 g a day.
- To stabilize moodiness and support relaxation, take 200 mg magnesium glycinate twice a day.
- To help improve sleep, take 100 to 200 mg L-theanine at night before bed.
- For general vitamin support, take daily:
  - Vitamin B_{12}, 1,000 mcg under the tongue
  - Biotin, 500 to 1,000 mcg
  - Vitamin B_6, 25 to 50 mg
  - Vitamin C, 500 to 1,000 mg
  - Vitamin D_3, 20 to 50 mcg

Exercise: You might think that a person who has trouble slowing down would do well with a calming exercise, but actually faster-paced exercises are more appropriate because they help "burn off the steam." Regularly incorporate at least a half hour of physical activity into your day. Two to three times a week try cycling, hiking, pick-up basketball, or an aerobics class. Jogging is also wonderful, but if you jog, start slowly and don't forget to stretch before and after your run.

Special Strategies: Pay attention to your sleep habits. Remember to turn off the television at least an hour before bed, and make sure that there is no ambient light in your room at all, not even a night-light. After dinner, take a long bath with lavender essential oil and drink a calming tea.

TYPE V: EXPLOSIVE, CAN'T SLOW DOWN

Profile: I once worked in the same hospital as a general surgeon who could have been a poster child for Type V SuperStress. He invariably scheduled two days' worth of work into every twenty-four hours, and then wondered why he crashed and burned at the end of the week. He had a reputation for quickly losing patience with anyone who didn't agree with him, which is surely why so many nurses refused to work with him. There are many people in this world of all occupations who are Type Vs: people in whom SuperStress creates aggressive behavior and a lack of resilience when they need it most. Type Vs essentially use every means possible to keep things going at an ultrafast pace—they live on coffee, caffeine-enhanced colas, or other stimulant-providing, sugar-laden foods. SuperStress creates a situation in which these people have little tolerance for mistakes, and when mistakes do occur, they often provoke an explosive reaction. Does this profile describe you? If so, understand that life doesn't have to remain this way. There are steps toward tranquility that you can begin to take right now.

Diet: Calm. That's your order of the day. And yes, you can eat your way to a less chaotic existence if you put your mind to it. Ideally a simple Mediterranean-style diet, with seafood (salmon, tuna, trout, sardines) as the protein source and whole grains for carbohydrates, will do the trick. If you're a sugar or caffeine "addict," now is the time to start weaning yourself. But whatever you do, don't go off caffeine cold turkey, because the withdrawal effects are very unpleasant. The best way to wean yourself from caffeine drinks (which include coffee, colas, and enery drinks) is this: If you are a five-cups-of-coffee-a-day person, for the first four days have only four cups. Then have three cups a day for the next three days and so on until you are off coffee completely. Let me add just a word about everyone's favorite substance: sugar. It's no secret that sugar acts as a quick fix, a.k.a. a *temporary* pick-me-up. If you're a true Type V, you have enough stimulation already, so kicking the sugar habit will only do you good. Start by replacing foods made with added sugar with foods that have natural sweeteners, such as honey or naturally sweetened ripe pineapple, bananas, and figs. Advance your sugar detox by limiting your dessert choices to berries and other fruits. There is plenty of natural sugar in many of the foods we eat, so if you become diligent about reading labels, you will be able to eliminate most added sugar. Try it for a week. You'll be amazed at how good you feel.

Supplements: You can help yourself out here, too. Try these as an addition to your diet.

- For anti-inflammatory support, take omega-3 fatty acid fish oil, 1 g a day.
- To stabilize moodiness and support relaxation, take 200 mg magnesium glycinate twice a day.
- To help improve sleep at night, take 100 to 200 mg L-theanine half an hour before bedtime.
- For general vitamin support, take daily:
  - Vitamin B_{12}, 1,000 mcg under the tongue
  - Biotin, 500 to 1,000 mcg
  - Vitamin B_6, 25 to 50 mg
  - Vitamin C, 500 to 1,000 mg
  - Vitamin D_3, 25 to 50 mcg

Exercise: Any physical activity is going to help you work off your anger and obsessive nature. In fact, that's the general idea. Take the edge off your pent-up emotions by letting them out. Running is a great way to do this. So are aerobics, biking, and even speed walking. If you have access to a gym, there are any number of machines that will allow you to surrender a lot of what's bothering you. For Type Vs, what's more important than the amount of time you spend at any activity is that you do *something* every day. No excuses about not having a block of time. You can split your activities into short segments if time is an issue for you. For ways to do it, see my exercise prescription plan in Chapter 5.

Special strategies: For you, there is perhaps nothing more grounding than a vigorous hike in the woods or as close as you can come to one. Try your local arboretum, a park, even your neighborhood streets. Go early in the morning. Stop every so often and close your eyes. Listen to the sounds of the birds or a running stream. Inhale the scents of the trees and morning dew on the grass. Another way to calm yourself is a nice relaxing massage or Reiki treatment. Try one. Try both. It can't hurt, and will surely help.

SYMPTOM SOLUTIONS

Not everyone will see themselves in the type profiles. Many of you will simply want to start slowly and approach one SuperStress symptom at a time. Toward that end, I offer here my integrative medicine chest— the herbs, essential oils, and other treatments I often prescribe for patients. I suggest you try them under the supervision of a qualified healthcare provider.

A word of caution, though. Although I've focused the majority of recommendations for each symptom on botanicals and supplements, I can't emphasize enough how important it is to pay attention to your lifestyle, too. You can't just take the right herbs and supplements and expect to feel better. You need to pay attention to all the elements in your life. For the best results, stay hydrated by drinking enough water, engage in some sort of physical activity, and practice mind/body exercises.

Herbs

Herbs (also known as botanicals) sold as over-the-counter dietary supplements are regulated as foods. The dosing is not uniform among manufacturers, but there are dosing suggestions on each manufacturer's label. Botanicals are sold in many forms: fresh or dried products, liquid or solid extracts, tablets, capsules, powders, or tea bags. For example, fresh ginger root is often found in the produce section of food stores but can also be found as a liquid or solid extract, as a tea or in capsules. Often a particular group of chemicals or a single chemical may be isolated from a botanical and identified on the supplement label. These isolated chemicals are often referred to as active principles or constituents. If you want to verify dosing and seek more information on any herbal preparation, you can easily access the American Botanical Council website (http://abc.herbalgram.org) or the National Institutes of Health website on dietary supplements (http://ods.od.nih.gov/factsheets/botanicalbackground.asp). Both of these sources are recognized as reputable references.

Anxiety

Anxiety is a response to perceived danger or psychological stress. It's a normal fear response, but if unaddressed for too long, it can develop into a disorder. Anxiety is, in fact, the most common of all mood disorders. If your anxiety is at the level of a disorder, you may find that engaging in talk or cognitive therapy is useful and lends insight about how the problem emerged in the first place. But you don't have to wait to have a diagnosed disorder to seek therapy. My suggestions should help at any stage along the anxiety spectrum.

It is important to remove all stimulants (caffeine, sugar, and so on) from your diet and to bolster the presence of omega-3 fatty acids. You can do this by eating salmon, sardines, or herring two or three times a week. If you're just not a fish lover, you can add 1 to 3 grams of omega-3 fatty acid fish oil to your daily supplement intake or 1 to 3 grams of flaxseed oil.

Breath work is one of the most powerful ways to address anxiety in an acute situation and is a portable form of calming your nervous system. There are lots of ways to do this and four of them can be found in Chapter 3. Acupuncture and massage are other strategies that can help your body remember its natural relaxation response—even if it hasn't visited it in years. Find a licensed practitioner today!

Supplements: Take one or more of the following daily.

- Magnesium 200 to 400 mg or a calcium-magnesium combination (1000 mg of calcium and 400 mg of magnesium)
- L-theanine 100 to 200 mg
- Vitamin D$_3$ 25 to 50 mcg

Herbal Tea: Brew a cup made with any of the following herbs and enjoy several times a day. The easiest way to do this is to use a liquid extract, placing 10 to 15 drops of any of these in a cup of warm water:

- Hops (*Humulus lupulus*)
- Kava (*Piper methysticum*)
- Linden (*Tilia cordata* Miller)
- Baical skullcap (*Scutellaria baicalensis*)
- Passion flower (*Passiflora incarnata*)
- Valerian (*Valeriana officinalis*)
- Holy basil (*Ocimum sanctum*)

Depression

Depression, the second most common mood disorder, can be mild, moderate, or severe. A regular sleep-wake cycle (awake at 7:00 A.M. and asleep by 11:00 P.M.) and aerobic exercise are two excellent ways to use lifestyle modification to stabilize depression's physical effects.

Try thirty minutes of aerobic exercise three to four times a week to start. If your depression is worse in the winter, it may respond to a full-spectrum light. Employ light therapy in the morning for ten to twenty minutes with a light intensity of 10,000 lux. *Lux* is the measure of brightness of the light; think of it as the dose of light intensity required to help seasonal affective disorder. In addition, you may want to consider daily meditation, and perhaps counseling as well.

Supplements: The following supplements are designed for *mild* depression. Moderate or severe depression should be managed in conjunction with a healthcare or mental health professional. Use *only one* of these three.

- Saint-John's-wort (*Hypericum perforatum*), standardized to .3 percent hypericin or 2 to 4 percent hyperforin: Take 900 mg per day in equally divided doses.
- S-adenosyl methionine (SAMe): Take 400 mg twice a day.
- 5-HTP: Start at 50 mg three times a day, then increase to 100 mg three times a day. *Don't use with Saint-John's-wort or any of the supplements mentioned in this section with any conventional depression medication without medical supervision.*

Supplements: Take these supplements daily:

- Vitamin B_{12}, 1,000 mcg under the tongue
- Vitamin B_6, 25 to 50 mg
- Omega-3 fatty acid fish oil, 3 g
- Vitamin D_3, 25 to 50 mcg
- Inositol, 1 to 4 g

Chronic Fatigue Syndrome (CFS)

A diagnosis of CFS includes medically unexplained fatigue of at least six months' duration that is not due to exercise, is not relieved by rest, and interferes with daily activities. It also includes at least four of the following: poor memory of recent events, sore throat, tender lymph nodes, muscle pain, pain in more than one joint without swelling, headaches, nonrefreshing sleep, and persistent feeling of illness for at least twenty-four hours after exercise. The onset of CFS in people with SuperStress generally follows an intense period of hard work and stress. Sometimes it can be aggravated by a flulike viral episode or psychologically traumatic event. The definitive reasons for chronic fatigue have yet to be determined, but the symptoms are very real. There are a number of factors that account for the symptoms of CFS. Each person with a diagnosis of CFS will have a distinctive pattern to their fatigue. Though the following suggestions may seem lengthy, there are so many options because there are many things to rebalance and restore. If you think you are experiencing CFS as a result of SuperStress, here is what I recommend.

Supplements: For building up energy, take L-carnitine, up to 3 g a day in capsule form, and add *one* of the following:

- Eleuthero (*Eleutherococcus senticosus*): Take 2 to 3 g in capsule form a day. Note that it can elevate blood pressure.
- Ginseng (*Panax ginseng*): Take 400 mg to 1 g a day. Note: That can elevate blood pressure.
- American ginseng (*Panax quinquefolius* L): Take 1 to 3 g of dried powder a day. Note that it can elevate blood pressure.
- *Rhodiola rosea:* Take 100 to 300 mg a day in capsule form.

For a late-afternoon pick-me-up, enjoy:

- Maté tea (*Ilex paraguariensis*)
- Licorice tea: Note that licorice tea, like the above energy boosters, can elevate blood pressure.
- Dark chocolate: one ounce a day is a great energizing snack, and it's excellent for an afternoon energy booster.

Other supporting strategies include:

- Acupuncture on a regular basis.
- Immune-building herbs such as *Astragalus;* take 4 to 7 g a day in capsule form.
- Medicinal mushrooms, such as shiitake (take 1 to 5 g in capsule form a day) and Reishi (take 1 to 1.5 g in capsule form a day).
- Maitake mushrooms (*Grifola frondosa*): Take 3 g a day in capsule form.
- Vitamin D_3: Take 25 to 50 mcg a day.
- Vitamin B_6: Take 25 to 50 mg a day.
- Vitamin B_{12}: Take 1,000 mcg a day under the tongue.
- Take 600 mg Malic acid twice a day. It helps stabilize the muscles.
- Take 100 mg alpha lipoic acid a day. It is an antioxidant and liver-support vitamin.

Gastric Distress/Irritable Bowel Syndrome

I can't count how many people with SuperStress also experience irritable bowel syndrome (IBS) and its uncomfortable symptoms, but my estimate would be one out of every four people. Because the brain has a direct effect on the gut, the stomach has always been one of the primary places where stress shows up. Foods that start the IBS cycle differ with each person, so if you suffer from IBS, I suggest you keep a food journal for a week. Jot down what you eat and when your symptoms occur. Also, note the non-food-related circumstances that you think contribute to your stress. Keeping a journal for a week will help you figure out which foods and situations are suspect. Then you can try to avoid them and see what happens.

If you are suffering from stress-related IBS, any of the mind/body exercises in Chapter 3 will be helpful to you.

Supplements: The following supplements will help relieve your symptoms.

- Fennel (*Foeniculum vulgare* Mill): Take 2 to 5 g in tea form two to four times per day.
- Glutamine: a nonessential amino acid that helps build up the microenvironment of the intestinal system; take 1 to 8 g per day.
- Probiotics (*lactobacillus, acidophilus*): Take 10 billion CFU (colony-forming units) per day on an empty stomach.
- Enteric-coated peppermint capsules can be taken with meals for cramps.

IMMUNE SYSTEM SUPPORT

SuperStressed individuals are highly vulnerable to viral illnesses. So, to boost your immune system during highly stressful times, I suggest a daily dose of the following.

- *Astragalus* dry root: 4 to 7 g or Ashwagandha (*Withania somnifera*): 3 to 6 g
- Vitamin D_3 (cholecalciferol): 25 to 50 mcg
- Maitake mushroom (*Grifola frondosa*): 1 g dried powder twice a day
- If you are suffering from a viral illness, try elderberry (*Sambucus nigra*); take 1 teaspoon of elderberry syrup per day. Sometimes the dose varies among manufacturers, so be sure to first check the label. (Sambucol, Nature's Way)

Insomnia

Some of these suggestions are found in my sleep prescription on page 99, and I advise you to visit it again. But here are a few of the more essential tips:

First and foremost, remove all stimulants from your diet. This includes coffee, nonherbal tea, caffeinated colas, or in fact any soda that has the word *caffeine* on the label. Chocolate has caffeine and other stimulants in it, too, so if you want to be a real purist, you're going to have to forgo the small piece of chocolate that's left on your pillow in all those fancy hotels—or at least save it until morning. If you're not physically active, start an exercise routine *but not within three hours of bedtime.* Create an evening ritual that cues your body that you're winding down.

Supplements:
- Melatonin: Take 1 to 3 mg thirty minutes before bed.
- For more assistance in falling asleep, add 100 mg L-theanine 30 minutes before bed.

Libido Support

Loss of libido is a complicated but commonly reported difficulty for both men and women, and SuperStress can cause or exacerbate the issue. Certain medicines and substances suppress libido. These include alcohol, antidepressants, and certain antihypertensives. Working with a urologist in conjunction with a psychotherapist or sex therapist is helpful. But these supplements may also help. Choose *only one.*

- Maca (*Lepidium meyenii*): Take 1,500 to 3,000 mg a day.
- Yohimbe (*Pausinystalia yohimbe*): Take 15 to 30 mg a day.
  Note: Watch blood pressure.

Memory Support for "Tired Brain Syndrome"

Scattered attention and poor memory (aka "Tired Brain Syndrome") are very commonly reported in symptoms of SuperStress. Emotional turmoil, multitasking, overloading the day, and overstimulation contribute to the problem. For any of these issues I suggest the following supplements, all three of which may be taken together if you choose.

- Phosphatidylcholine: Take 500 mg a day in equally divided doses.
- Phosphatidylserine: Take 100 mg three times a day.
- Huperzine A: Take 50 to 200 mcg a day.

PMS

Premenstrual syndrome affects 20 to 50 percent of women. The intensity of symptoms varies from woman to woman but is worsened by SuperStress. Symptoms can begin a few hours or up to fourteen days prior to the onset of menses. Physical symptoms include backache, bloating, breast fullness, fatigue, hot flashes, insomnia, lack of energy, swelling of hands and feet, and cramps. Mood changes include agitation, confusion, crying spells, depression, difficulty concentrating, emotional hypersensitivity, forgetfulness, mood swings, nervousness, and social withdrawal. I have had moderate success with my patients (some, but not all, do very well) using the following supplements.

- Calcium: 1,000 to 1,500 mg a day
- Evening primrose: 2 to 4 g a day
- Vitex (*Vitex agnus-castus*): 500 mg to 1 g three times a day
- Magnesium glycinate: 200 mg a day

Essential Oils

Essential oils can be used in addition to any of the supplements listed above. I favor essential oils because they are easy to find, portable, and often very effective. One of the reasons oils are so effective in mind/body situations is that the olfactory system generates signals directly to the brain area that affects emotion, the limbic system. Some small clinical studies have indicated that it takes very few molecules of these essential oils to create a mood effect. The best way to use essential oils is to add two or three drops to a teaspoonful of a neutral oil like canola, and place the oil in a diffuser. A diffuser dispenses the essential oil; they range from a simple ceramic dish to an electric-powered mechanism. The object is for the oil to slowly vaporize into the air. Another way to dispense oil is to add three to fifteen drops to a warm bath, or add ten drops per ounce to massage oil. *Never ingest essential oils or apply them directly to the skin.* Studies show that the following oils may be beneficial for the conditions listed.

Anxiety
- Chamomile
- Pine
- Rose
- Ylang-ylang

Insomnia
- Cedar
- Lavender
- Sandalwood

Stress/overwork
- Chamomile
- Eucalyptus
- Juniper
- Lavender

All of these remedies work for the stress-related problems outlined above, but for those suffering from more than one of these diagnoses, it's worth remembering that the four-week-program, although more involved, may be ultimately more lasting in helping you manage your problems. The reason, of course, is that SuperStress usually needs a multilayered intervention—lifestyle changes *plus* any of the above suggested solutions pertinent to the specific problem or problems.

Final Thoughts

LIVING SERENITY

I WOULD LIKE TO CONGRATULATE YOU for your perseverance and integrity in stepping up to the plate to explore a different way to negotiate life—it's not easy to look in the mirror and realize that things aren't what they used to be and that change is required.

But you did it.

You showed up and had faith in yourself.

My hope was to provide you with enough information and perspective on the integrative process so that you could shape it to fit your needs. The plan's effectiveness lies in your ability to regularly do the things you have set out to achieve.

Every change has cycles or periodicity. What goes up also comes down, when there is day there is night, and so on. Likewise, when there is change there is also the potential of failure. Or at least that is how people interpret it when they reach an obstacle for the first time. That's a natural response to change. What is occurring is that your "old self" is learning what it feels like to be your "new self" by observing contrast. If by some chance you temporarily step off the plan and reenter your old discomfort zone, I have good news for you . . . you now know just how good it feels to be in control of your life and my guess is that you'll want to have that feeling again. When you step back on the plan, and I know you will, this time it will feel more familiar because you've been through it before.

This is your ultimate lesson about the Four-Week SuperStress Solution Program. It's a flexible plan. The success of this program is not in its rigid perfection of execution but in its fluidity to fit with your life.

I've given you lots of messages throughout this book. I have shared my life stories and those of my patients. You've been with me to Micronesia and back. Through it all I suppose if I had to give you one last message on how best to handle SuperStress, it would be to reach out to someone else. As Arthur Pine, the father of a good friend, put it, "Caring can start a domino effect."[1] Reach out and reach far. Do something kind for someone or help someone out. Reaching out to help someone reminds us of the interconnected nature of the human experience and our capacity to aspire to be the very best we can be—something we often forget.

Appendix

REGULAR MENUS

HERE ARE TWO WEEKS' WORTH—fourteen days—of "regular" meal plans, menus for you to follow (or adapt) during weeks one, three, and four of the four-week-program. All recipes yield one portion unless otherwise stated. Note that any shake can be made with any milk, but I favor unsweetened almond milk because it has the lowest calorie content.

DAY 1

Breakfast

PROTEIN SHAKE
>1 cup plain yogurt—live culture, low fat
>1 tsp vanilla extract
>1 cup blueberries
>2 tsp honey
>½ cup mint (peppermint)—fresh if possible
>1 tbsp ground flaxseed
>1 tbsp wheat germ
>½ cup low-fat milk or ½ cup almond, soy, or skim milk
>Optional: 2 tbsp whey, hemp, or rice-protein powder

>*Or*

STEEL-CUT OATS
>¾ cup cooked in ⅓ cup low-fat milk or almond milk
>1 tbsp ground flaxseed (add right at the end) and 1 tbsp wheat germ
>2 tsp honey or brown sugar

>Coffee or tea

Mid-Morning Snack

1 Apple

Lunch

2 cups romaine lettuce or mixed greens
¼ cup pregrated or chopped carrots, or mini carrot sticks
¼ cup cherry tomatoes
2 oz lean turkey, chicken, ham, or tofu
Optional: ¼ avocado, sliced, or 1 ounce cheese
Dressing: juice of ½ lemon, 2 tbsp olive oil, 2 sprinkles of Mrs. Dash
   seasoning

Afternoon Snack

1 apple or ⅓ dark chocolate bar
Tea

MASIE'S MOM'S INCREDIBLE TEA
For a treat during this week or any other part of the diet, try this delicious tea!

Take an airtight tin of your favorite loose tea (rooibos tea infusion or Ceylon tea work well) and add ½ cup of dried cherries to the tea leaves. The taste is stronger the longer the cherries are kept with the tea. When you brew the tea, make sure to get a few cherries in the cup. The cherries are delicious to eat after you've brewed your tea. Add a splash of milk and some almond or vanilla extract if desired. This is a great tea before bed.

If you need a quick fix you can add a small amount of cherry preserves to a cup of tea for a sweet, fast treat.

Dinner

1 cup miso soup (1 to 2 tsp golden miso in 1 cup of hot water)
1 cup cooked brown rice
2 cups steamed Brussels sprouts
Lentils Plus

LENTILS PLUS
    ½ cup cooked lentils
    2 garlic cloves, ground
    ½ tsp curry powder
    1½ cups cilantro, chopped
    ½ onion
    ½ cup water
    2 cups lightly chopped vegetables from the following: onions, carrots,
        tomatoes, bell peppers, peas
    Optional: ½ chicken bouillon cube (dissolved in the water)
    ½ tsp mustard seed

Sauté the lentils with the garlic, curry powder, cilantro, and onion, then braise until soft in ½ cup of water, with or without bouillon added. Add the vegetables and, if desired, mustard seed.

Dessert

BAKED PEAR
    1 pear
    2 tbsp red wine
    2 tbsp water
    Zest of ½ lemon
    1 tbsp sugar
    ½ stick cinnamon or 1 tsp ground cinnamon

Peel, core, and slice the pear. Place ingredients in a covered baking dish. Bake at 375 degrees for 1 hour.
    Adapted from *Julia Child's Kitchen*[1]

DAY 2

Breakfast

    1½ cup Kashi cereal with 1 cup almond milk or skim milk
    1 cup berries (blueberries, blackberries, strawberries, or raspberries)

    Or

    2 slices Egg White Frittata

EGG WHITE FRITTATA
SERVES 8 TO 10

> ½ tbsp olive oil
>
> 10 cups packed spinach or arugula leaves
>
> 2 cloves finely chopped garlic
>
> 2 chopped scallions (white and green parts)
>
> 8 beaten eggs or 10 egg white equivalents
>
> 1 oz Parmesan cheese (grated)
>
> ½ tsp chopped fresh herbs (rosemary, thyme, oregano, sage) or 1 tsp dried herbs
>
> Optional: 1 tsp lemon zest

Preheat oven to 325 degrees. In a large skillet, combine olive oil, spinach leaves, garlic, and scallions. Lightly cook for 3 to 5 minutes. Drain off liquid.

In a bowl, add eggs to cooked spinach mixture and add Parmesan cheese and herbs. In a 9-inch ovenproof pan, spray olive oil on surface to lightly coat and pour in the mixture. Bake at 325 degrees for 25 to 30 minutes until eggs are golden and set.

> Coffee or tea

Mid-Morning Snack

> ⅓ cup almonds
>
> 1 apple

Lunch

> 1 cup of bean salad
>
> 4 rice crackers with 1 tbsp of nut butter spread

BEAN SALAD

> ½ cup kidney beans
>
> ½ cup garbanzo beans
>
> 2 green onions, finely chopped
>
> ⅓ cup cherry tomatoes
>
> ½ cup parsley, finely chopped

Mix with 1 tbsp of Dr. Lee's Famous Salad Dressing

DR. LEE'S FAMOUS SALAD DRESSING
4 tbsp olive oil
1 tbsp rice wine vinegar
1 tsp Dijon mustard
1 tsp honey
½ clove garlic, minced
A sprinkle of Mrs. Dash seasoning
Optional: Minced basil, oregano, or thyme to taste

Afternoon Snack

1 cup of dried cherries
⅓ bar of dark chocolate
Tea

Dinner

3 oz grilled breast of chicken with sliced lemon and grilled Vidalia
onion on top
1 cup brown rice
1 cup peas
Salad of romaine lettuce, cherry tomatoes, sliced apple, and toasted
pine nuts with Dr. Lee's Famous Salad Dressing (see above)

Dessert

ORANGE WITH WALNUTS
1 navel orange, peeled and sliced
2 tbsp crushed walnuts
3 tbsp honey

Mix walnuts, honey, and orange slices. For garnish add a sprig of spearmint.

DAY 3

Breakfast

PROTEIN SHAKE
  ½ cup almond milk, skim milk, light soy milk, or rice milk
  1 nectarine or 1 cup peaches, fresh or frozen
  2 tbsp shredded coconut
  2 tbsp whey protein powder
  1 cup plain low-fat yogurt
  ½ tsp vanilla extract

  Or

  2 slices Egg White Frittata (see page 234)

  Or

  1 ½ cups Kashi cereal with 1 cup almond or skim milk

  Coffee or tea

Mid-Morning Snack

  ⅓ cup dried cranberries, currants, or cherries
  ¼ cup almonds
  1 apple

Lunch

  2 turkey meatballs (see recipe below)

  Or

  ¼ cup hummus
  2 cups total mixed baby carrots, sliced bell pepper, celery, and cherry
      tomatoes
  ½ avocado drizzled with lemon juice
  1 Pita bread

TURKEY MEATBALLS

MAKES 6 MEATBALLS

    1 lb ground turkey

    1 egg

    ½ cup seasoned bread crumbs

    1 tsp chopped onions

    ¼ tsp garlic powder

    ⅛ tsp black pepper

    1 tbsp tomato paste or 2 tbsp ketchup

Preheat oven to 400 degrees. Combine all the ingredients and mix thoroughly. Form meatballs from 1 tbsp of mixture, and mold into the shape of a ball. Bake 15 to 20 minutes on a lightly oiled 10 x 15 x 1 inch pan, or until the meatballs are no longer pink in the center.

Note: This recipe yields more meatballs than just two, but it's so good you might want to share it with friends or save half of the meatballs in the freezer for another meal.

Afternoon Snack

    1 orange

    ⅓ cup shelled sunflower seeds

    Tea

Dinner

    4 oz salmon, broiled, with thinly sliced sautéed onion on top and slivers of thin-sliced lemon

    1 medium baked potato plus ½ tsp butter

    1 cup steamed broccoli; topped with 1 tsp grated Parmesan cheese

    1 cup steamed asparagus, drizzled with 1 tsp olive oil and ½ clove garlic, finely minced, and minced thyme and oregano

Dessert

    2 kiwi fruit

    ¾ cup vanilla yogurt

DAY 4

Breakfast

PROTEIN SHAKE

¼ cup each of blueberries, peaches, strawberries, banana slices

2 tbsp whey protein powder

1 cup plain low-fat yogurt

½ cup of almond or skim milk

1 tsp vanilla

Or

2 slices whole wheat toast

1 organic egg, cooked any way you like

½ grapefruit

Coffee or tea

Mid-Morning Snack

2 rice cakes with 2 tbsp almond butter

Lunch

Tuna Salad Sandwich

½ cup baby carrots

⅓ cup almonds

1 apple

TUNA SALAD SANDWICH

3 oz water-packed tuna

2 tbsp mayonnaise or Dijon mustard

¼ tsp mustard powder (omit if adding Dijon mustard)

¼ tsp curry powder

2 tbsp diced celery

2 tsp diced onion

2 slices tomato

1 lettuce leaf or small handful of alfalfa sprouts
2 slices whole wheat bread

Afternoon Snack

1 medium-size pear or 1 apple
Tea

Dinner

Beet Green Medley
Salad

BEET GREEN MEDLEY
SERVES 2

3 beets with greens (tops)
1 cup sliced shiitake mushrooms
1 cup cherry tomatoes
½ onion, sliced
1 block of firm or baked tofu (20 oz)

Chop and stir-fry beet greens. Stir-fry the beets with the rest of the vegetables and the tofu in 2 tbsp of olive oil and add 3 slices of fresh ginger root. Sprinkle with soy sauce. Serve with 1 cup of brown rice.

SALAD

½ cup golden raisins
2 cups grated carrots
1 tsp lemon juice
1 tsp grated ginger
1 tsp olive oil

Mix all ingredients together.

Dessert

½ cantaloupe

DAY 5

Breakfast

SHAKE

½ cup water, or almond, low-fat soy, or skim milk

½ cup tofu (optional; great for women over forty-five because it is a natural source of plant-based phytoestrogens)

2 tsp honey

2 tbsp wheat germ

½ cup apricot, strawberries, peaches, or 2 peeled kiwi fruit

Or

2 slices of the frittata

2 slices of whole wheat toast with one pat butter

Coffee or tea

Mid-Morning Snack

⅓ cup almonds

Lunch

Black Bean Spread sandwich

1 banana

⅓ cup almonds or hazelnuts

BLACK BEAN SPREAD

MAKES 1½ CUPS

1 cup black beans

2 tbsp tomato paste

1 tsp basil (fresh, if possible)

2 tsp rice wine vinegar or balsamic vinegar

1 small stalk celery, chopped

½ tsp garlic powder

Optional: ½ tsp cumin

Mix the ingredients in a blender until they reach the consistency of crunchy peanut butter.

For a sandwich, spread over 1 or 2 slices of whole wheat toast, and top with cucumber slices, tomato slices, and alfalfa sprouts or lettuce. Add 1 slice of low-fat cheese if you wish.

Afternoon Snack

1 apple
⅓ cup of dates
Tea

Dinner

Trout Surprise
Baked sweet potato
Cucumber salad

TROUT SURPRISE

Preheat oven to 400 degrees. Wrap in foil or parchment baking paper: 1 medium size rainbow trout. Stuff cavity with thin slices of onion and lemon. Rub outside of fish with ½ tsp olive oil. Season lightly with thyme; salt and pepper to taste. Bake for 25 minutes or until tender.

CUCUMBER SALAD

SERVES 2

½ cup rice wine vinegar
½ tsp sugar
1 cucumber, peeled and sliced

Mix the vinegar and sugar; marinate the cucumber slices in the mixture for several hours. Serve at room temperature or chilled.

Dessert

1 (2-inch) slice angel food cake with ½ cup strawberries sweetened with
    1 tsp sugar

DAY 6

Breakfast

SMOOTHIE
    1 banana
    1 tsp peanut butter
    ½ cup low-fat, soy, almond, or skim milk
    2 tsp honey
    1 cup plain low-fat yogurt

Or

    ¾ cup steel-cut oats cooked in ⅓ cup low-fat or almond milk
    1 tbsp ground flaxseed and 1 tbsp wheat germ (added after cooking)
    2 tsp honey or brown sugar

    Coffee or tea

Mid-Morning Snack

    4 rye crackers with 2 tbsp almond butter

Lunch

POCKET PITA SANDWICH
    ¼ cup olives
    ¼ cup avocado
    4 slices of cucumber
    3 slices of tomato
    ⅓ cup carrots
    1 tbsp of Tahini Salad Dressing

Mix the vegetables together in a bowl with the Tahini Salad Dressing.
Place all in pita.

TAHINI SALAD DRESSING
MAKES 1½ CUPS
>   ½ cup tahini
>   ½ cup olive oil
>   juice of 1 lemon
>   ½ cup water
>   1 tbsp soy sauce
>   Optional: 1 clove garlic or ½ tsp garlic powder and sprinkle of hot
>   pepper flakes

Afternoon Snack

>   ⅓ dark chocolate bar
>   Tea

Dinner

ASIAN NOODLE DINNER SALAD
SERVES 2
>   1 broiled 3 oz breast of chicken, shredded, or 3 oz of deveined cooked
>   shrimp
>   2 cups chopped romaine lettuce
>   ½ cup cherry tomatoes
>   2 scallions, sliced (both white and green parts)
>   3 tbsp chopped cilantro
>   ½ cup snow peas
>   2 or 3 tbsp of Asian Dressing
>
>   Noodles
>   1 16-ounce package of thin Chinese noodles or Soba noodles or angel
>   hair pasta

Take a quarter of the package of noodles for each serving and place in boiling water for 3 to 4 minutes. Cook only until just soft (*al dente*) but not too soft; separate the strands while boiling. Drain in colander and immediately rinse with cold water. Cool noodles in the refrigerator. Mix with other ingredients and dressing.

ASIAN DRESSING
    3 tbsp dark sesame oil
    3 tbsp soy sauce (light)
    2 tbsp balsamic or rice wine vinegar
    2 tbsp sugar
    1 tbsp peanut butter
    2 tbsp grated ginger
    Zest of ½ lemon
    ½ tsp garlic powder

Dessert

    1 cup blueberries

DAY 7

Breakfast

PROTEIN SHAKE
    ½ cup orange juice
    1 cube of soft tofu or 1 tbsp whey or rice protein powder
    1 banana
    ¼ tsp vanilla extract
    1 tbsp of wheat germ
    2 tbsp ground flaxseed

    Or

    1 whole wheat muffin
    1 tbsp peanut butter
    1 medium banana

    Coffee or tea

Mid-Morning Snack

    8 rice crackers and 1 oz of cheese

Lunch

2 cups low-fat pea soup

8 rice crackers

Cucumber/tomato salad: mix of ½ cucumber (skinned) and sliced, ½
cup cherry tomatoes, 1 tbsp olive oil, and 1 tsp lemon juice

ADELE'S LOW-CAL PEA SOUP

SERVES 2

1 9 oz package of frozen peas

2 cups hot water

1 cube chicken or vegetable bouillon

Optional: 2 tbsp fresh spearmint

Dash of salt to taste

Mix all ingredients in a blender until smooth. Serve cold, or heat in the
microwave 1 to 2 minutes.

Sprinkle red pepper flakes for zing, if you like.

Afternoon Snack

1 apple

Tea

Dinner

Chinese Halibut

Green Mashed Potatoes

Salad

CHINESE HALIBUT

4 oz of baked or broiled halibut

½ tsp soy sauce

1 tbsp grated ginger

½ tsp minced garlic

1 tsp olive oil

Preheat oven to 400 degrees. Place the halibut in the center of a piece of alu-
minum foil. Season the fish with soy sauce, ginger, garlic, and olive oil. Pinch
the foil closed. Bake for 8 to 10 minutes until fish is cooked through.

GREEN MASHED POTATOES
Boil 1 peeled medium-sized potato. Place in food processor with ⅓ package (9 to 10 oz) spinach. Blend, heat, and serve.

SALAD
Drizzle tomato slices with olive oil and sprinkle with ¼ cup minced purple onion.

Dessert

2 cups air-popped popcorn

Or

2 tangerines

DAY 8

Breakfast

SMOOTHIE
1 banana
½ cup pineapple (canned or fresh)
½ cup almond or soy milk, orange juice, or water
2 tbsp protein powder
1 tbsp wheat germ
1 tbsp dried coconut flakes

Or

¾ cup steel-cut oats cooked in ⅓ cup low-fat or almond milk
1 tbsp ground flaxseed (add at the end)
1 tbsp wheat germ
2 tsp honey or brown sugar

Coffee or tea

Mid-Morning Snack

4 rye crisp crackers with 2 tbsp cashew butter

Lunch

¼ cup hummus
2 cups cut vegetables (celery sticks, cucumber, radishes, bell pepper,
    mini carrots, cherry tomatoes)
3 oz of ham or chicken or turkey
1 apple

Afternoon Snack

⅓ dark chocolate bar
Tea
Optional: 2 graham crackers

Dinner

Pasta with Pesto and Shrimp
Salad of 1 cup of baby arugula with 2 tbsp sliced Parmesan cheese and
    Raspberry Vinegar Dressing

PASTA WITH PESTO AND SHRIMP

1 cup cooked whole wheat spaghetti or spinach fettuccine
2 tbsp pesto sauce
6 shrimp (deveined and shelled)
1 tbsp olive oil
½ chopped onion
¼ cup peas

Stir fry the shrimp with the olive oil, onion, and peas. Mix in the noodles and dress with the pesto.

RASPBERRY VINEGAR DRESSING
  1 tbsp raspberry vinegar
  2 tbsp olive oil
  ½ clove garlic, minced
  1 tsp basil
  ½ tsp oregano
  ½ tsp thyme

Mix all ingredients thoroughly.

Dessert

  1 cup strawberries sweetened with 1 tsp sugar

DAY 9

Breakfast

SMOOTHIE
  ⅓ cup Açaí berry pulp (look for this in any health food store's frozen
      food section)
  ½ cup almond, soy, or skim milk
  1 tsp honey
  1 tbsp ground flaxseed
  1 tbsp wheat germ
  ½ banana

  Or

  1½ cups Kashi cereal with 1 cup almond or skim milk

  Coffee or tea

Mid-Morning Snack

  1 banana

  Or

  ⅓ cup dried cranberries and ⅓ cup walnuts

Lunch

Vegetable and Cheese Sandwich
⅓ cup baby carrots

VEGETABLE AND CHEESE SANDWICH

2 slices whole wheat bread
Sliced cucumber
Sliced tomato
2 slices low-fat cheese
alfalfa sprouts or lettuce
3 oz chicken, beef, ham, or sliced baked tofu
Spread: Dijon mustard

Afternoon Snack

1 cup grapefruit sections
Tea

Dinner

Shrimp and Vegetable Medley
1 cup brown rice
1 steamed artichoke (dip for artichoke: olive oil, ⅓ tsp minced garlic,
    and juice of ½ lemon)

SHRIMP AND VEGETABLE MEDLEY
SERVES 2

½ cup white onion, chopped
⅓ cup shiitake mushrooms, sliced
1 cup diagonally cut celery
⅓ cup cashews
½ cup sliced bell pepper
8 shrimp, deveined and peeled

In a heated pan sauté the vegetables with 1 tbsp olive oil until crisp. Add the shrimp and continue sautéing until shrimp are pink and cooked through.

Dessert

⅓ cup dried apricots

DAY 10

Breakfast

SMOOTHIE
½ cup blueberries
½ cup blackberries
½ cup strawberries
½ cup almond, soy, hemp, or skim milk
2 tbsp whey or protein powder
2 tbsp honey
1 tbsp ground flaxseed

Or

¾ cup of steel-cut oats cooked in ⅓ cup low-fat or almond milk

Coffee or tea

Mid-Morning Snack

⅓ cup dried cherries and ⅓ cup almonds

Lunch

1 whole wheat burrito filled with ⅓ cup pinto beans, mashed, 3 oz
     grated low-fat cheese, 2 tbsp salsa, 1 tsp fresh chopped cilantro
⅓ cup carrot sticks or baby carrots
1 orange

Afternoon Snack

10 vanilla wafers
Tea

Dinner

1 corn on the cob (boiled)
3 oz of halibut, broiled
1 cup steamed broccoli sprinkled with 1 tsp grated Parmesan

HALIBUT

3 oz halibut
¼ cup olive oil
1 clove garlic, mashed
½ cup chopped cilantro
2 tsp cumin powder
1 tbsp fresh lime juice
½ tsp red pepper flakes

Coat fish on both sides prior to broiling with mixture of olive oil, cilantro, cumin powder, lime juice, red pepper flakes.

Dessert

BAKED APPLE

Core and peel the top of an apple. Sprinkle with brown sugar and cinnamon and add a few raisins in the center where the core was removed. Place in a microwave-safe dish, cover with cellophane wrap, and microwave for 2 to 3 minutes, until soft. You can also place it, covered, in an oven at 350 degrees for 15 to 20 minutes or until done.

DAY 11

Breakfast

SMOOTHIE

1 cup cranberry juice
½ cup strawberries
½ cup raspberries
2 tbsp whey protein powder
1 tbsp wheat germ
1 tbsp ground flaxseed

½ cup plain low-fat yogurt
½ cup ice
1 tsp honey

Or

1½ cups Kashi cereal with 1 cup of almond or skim milk

Coffee or tea

Mid-Morning Snack

1 tbsp peanut butter
8 graham crackers

Lunch

2 cups shredded red cabbage
¼ cup kidney beans
½ cup cherry tomatoes
1 oz grated fresh Parmesan cheese
2 tbsp pine nuts
2 oz sliced or diced turkey
1 tbsp Dr. Lee's Famous Salad Dressing
1 green onion, sliced (white and green parts)
1 slice rye bread
1 pear or 1 cup grapefruit sections

Afternoon Snack

1 apple

Dinner

Curry Coconut Stew
1 cup brown rice (optional: top with 2 tbsp cilantro, freshly minced)
Cucumber Salad (see page 241)

CURRY COCONUT STEW

SERVES 2

> 3 tbsp olive oil
> 2 cloves garlic, minced
> ½ tbsp black mustard seeds
> 2 tsp curry powder
> 2 tbsp dried coconut flakes
> 1 cup onion, chopped
> 1 cup frozen peas
> 1 cup quartered potatoes
> 1 cup sliced carrots
> ½ cup tomatoes, diced
> 1 cup cauliflower
> ¼ cup raisins
> ½ cup water
> 1 tsp salt

In a deep skillet or Dutch oven over medium high heat, heat olive oil. Add 2 cloves of garlic, minced. Then add black mustard seeds, curry powder, and dried coconut flakes. Sauté for several minutes. Add all at once: chopped onions, frozen peas, quartered potatoes, sliced carrots, diced tomatoes, cauliflower, raisins, water, and salt. Cook for 20 to 30 minutes or until potatoes are tender when poked by a fork.

CUCUMBER SALAD

See page 241 for recipe.

Dessert

> ½ cup low-sugar canned peaches

> *Or*

> 1 whole fresh sliced peach or nectarine

DAY 12

Breakfast

SMOOTHIE
> ½ cup sliced mangos (fresh or frozen)
> ½ cup crushed ice
> ½ cup almond, soy, hemp, or skim milk
> Optional: 1 cup low-fat vanilla yogurt

> *Or*

> ¾ cup steel-cut oats cooked in ⅓ cup low-fat or almond milk

> Coffee or tea

Mid-Morning Snack

> ½ cup celery sticks
> ½ cup baby carrots or carrot sticks

Lunch

TURKEY SANDWICH
> 2 slices whole wheat bread
> 3 oz baked turkey slices
> 2 tbsp low-fat mayonnaise
> 2 tomato slices
> ¼ avocado, sliced
> 1 romaine lettuce leaf

Afternoon Snack

> 1 cup air-popped popcorn

Dinner

> Dr. Lee's Red Wine Chicken Stew
> 1 cup brown rice or 1 cup of whole wheat fettucine
> ½ cup peas

DR LEE'S RED WINE CHICKEN STEW

SERVES 2

- 1 tbsp olive oil
- 2 cloves of garlic, mashed
- ½ cup chopped tomatoes
- 2 boneless chicken breasts
- 1 cup sliced onion
- 1 cup sliced mushrooms
- 1 cup full-bodied red wine
- 1 cup chicken stock (1 cup water plus ½ chicken or vegetable bouillon cube)
- ¼ tsp thyme

In a Dutch oven at medium heat, combine olive oil and garlic and sauté briefly. Then add tomatoes and cook for five minutes. Add chicken breasts, onion, mushrooms, wine, chicken stock, and thyme. Lower heat and cook for 40 to 50 minutes until chicken breasts are done.

Dessert

Sliced pear
½ oz crumbled blue cheese

DAY 13

Breakfast

SMOOTHIE

- ½ cup raspberries
- 1 banana
- ½ tsp vanilla extract
- 1 cup plain low-fat yogurt
- ½ cup ice
- ½ tsp fresh mint
- ½ cup almond or skim milk
- Optional: ½ tsp cocoa powder and 2 tsp honey

Or

¾ cup steel-cut oats cooked in ⅓ cup low-fat or almond milk

Coffee or tea

Mid-Morning Snack

1 oz Swiss cheese slices
6 rice crackers

Lunch

Low-fat Carrot Ginger Soup
1 slice whole wheat toast
1 cup blueberries or dried cranberries
1 apple

LOW-FAT CARROT GINGER SOUP
SERVES 2

1 package frozen carrots
1½ cups hot water
1 cube vegetable or chicken bouillon
½ cup skim milk
1 tsp ginger, grated
1 tsp honey

In a blender put 1 package of frozen carrots, hot water, 1 cube vegetable or chicken bouillon, skim milk, grated ginger, and honey. Puree and warm in microwave for 2 minutes.

Afternoon Snack

2 oz dark chocolate
Tea

Dinner

Chili

1 cup brown rice

3 cups collard green leaves that have been sautéed until tender with
2 tbsp of pesto, 1 medium chopped tomato, and ½ cup of sliced
yellow onion

CHILI

SERVES 2

1 tbsp olive oil

1 cup canned black beans

½ cup corn

½ cup tomatoes, diced

½ cup onions, sliced

½ cup bell peppers, diced

½ tsp chili power

½ tsp cumin

1 clove garlic, mashed

1 tsp oregano

½ tsp thyme

½ cup cilantro

½ tsp cayenne or ¼ tsp red pepper flakes (optional)

In a Dutch oven place the following: olive oil, canned black beans, corn, diced tomatoes, sliced onions, diced bell peppers, chili powder, cumin, garlic, oregano and thyme, and cilantro. (Optional: cayenne or red pepper flakes.) Cook for 1 hour.

Dessert

Cup of hot chocolate flavored with 1 tbsp honey and/or cinnamon.

DAY 14

Breakfast

SMOOTHIE

1 cup plain low-fat yogurt

1 tsp vanilla extract

1 cup blueberries
2 tsp honey
½ cup fresh mint or ⅛ tsp mint extract
1 tbsp ground flaxseed
1 tbsp wheat germ
½ cup almond, soy, skim, or hemp milk
Optional: 2 tbsp whey, hemp, or rice protein powder

Coffee or tea

Mid-Morning Snack

2 whole wheat Fig Newtons
Tea

Lunch

½ cup hummus
1 cup baby carrots
½ cup cherry tomatoes
½ cup bell peppers
4 rye crisps
1 cup berries
1 apple

Afternoon Snack

2 oz dark chocolate
Tea

Dinner

3 oz red snapper, broiled (top with 1 tsp olive oil, 1 tsp cilantro, 1 tsp
    green onion, and juice of ½ lemon before broiling)
1 cup whole wheat fettuccine with ½ tbsp pesto
1 cup steamed asparagus drizzled with olive oil and lemon juice

Dessert

DR. LEE'S MOCHA MERINGUE

SERVES 2

    1 cup powdered sugar

    1 tbsp cocoa

    ⅛ tsp cinnamon

    ½ tsp instant coffee powder

    4 egg whites

    ½ tsp vanilla

    ½ cup slivered almonds

    ¼ tsp salt

Preheat oven to 250 degrees. Lightly grease a cookie sheet. Sift powdered sugar, cocoa, coffee, and salt. Put dry mix and almonds in a blender—grind until it becomes a fine powder. Beat the egg whites and vanilla extract until stiff. Fold the powdered mix into the stiff egg whites. Drop meringue mix with a tablespoon onto cookie sheet. Bake for 2 to 3 hours, turn off the oven, leave meringues in oven for 20 minutes, then serve.

    Adapted from *The Moosewood Cookbook* by Mollie Katzen.[2]

The SuperStress Solution Detox Diet

DETOX, SHORT FOR DETOXIFICATION, is the body's natural, ongoing process of neutralizing or eliminating toxins from the body for health. Toxins are anything that can potentially harm body tissue. The body is constantly detoxifying itself from the waste products it naturally creates. These waste products can be harmful if they are not neutralized and disposed of. The liver is the main organ that facilitates the process. Once the liver accomplishes this, the waste is eliminated by way of four systems: the intestines, the kidneys, the skin, and the lungs.

Generally, a detox diet is a short-term diet. The one I have included on the following pages is designed to emphasize foods that provide the vitamins, nutrients, and antioxidants that the body needs for detoxification. This includes high-fiber foods and lots of water, which draw out and eliminate toxins by increasing the frequency of bowel movements and urination. *Staying hydrated is essential on any detox diet.* You should be consuming *at least* two quarts of water a day. If you are accustomed to consuming coffee every day, shifting your consumption to green tea during this week will cut down on your caffeine intake and boost your vitamin consumption at the same time. But be careful if you stop caffeine cold turkey. You might experience a headache due to caffeine withdrawal.

You will also note that there is not a lot of variety in this diet. I've done that purposely because this is a week of rest for your digestive system, and having the same thing every day for a week allows your GI tract to rest.

NOTE: Anyone considering a detox diet, particularly pregnant women or people with chronic diseases, should consult a qualified health professional and their medical doctor first. Continuing a detox diet for longer than one week may result in nutrient deficiencies.

BREAKFAST FRUIT SHAKES

Every day for breakfast, try one of these shakes. To boost the vitamin content, add 1 tbsp of a "green powder"—for instance, New Chapter's Berry Green or Barlean's Greens. Another option is to add 2 tbsp of pureed spinach to any of these drinks.

Drink a shake at breakfast and as your mid-morning and afternoon snacks, or substitute the snacks with a Pick-Me-Up Green Drink.

SHAKE 1
Blend together:
> 1 cup plain low-fat yogurt (live culture)
> 1 tsp vanilla extract
> 1 cup blueberries
> 2 tsp honey
> ½ cup fresh mint or ⅛ tsp mint extract
> 1 tbsp ground flaxseed
> 1 tbsp wheat germ
> ½ cup almond, soy, skim, or hemp milk
> Optional: 2 tbsp of whey, hemp, or rice protein powder

SHAKE 2
Blend together:
> ½ cup almond, skim, light soy, or rice milk
> 1 nectarine or 1 cup fresh or frozen peaches
> 2 tbsp whey protein powder
> 1 cup plain low-fat yogurt
> ½ tsp vanilla extract

SHAKE 3
Blend together:
> ¼ cup each of blueberries, peaches, strawberries, banana slices
> 2 tbsp whey protein powder
> 1 cup plain low-fat yogurt
> ½ cup almond, soy, or skim milk
> 1 tsp vanilla extract

SHAKE 4

Blend together:

> ⅓ cup Açaí berry pulp
>
> ½ cup almond, soy, or skim milk
>
> 1 tsp honey
>
> 1 tbsp ground flaxseed
>
> 1 tbsp wheat germ
>
> ½ banana

PICK-ME-UP GREEN DRINK FOR MID-MORNING
OR AFTERNOON SNACKS

Blend together:

> 1 large or two medium-size peeled Granny Smith apples
>
> 1 5-inch celery stalk, cut into segments
>
> 2 peeled kiwi
>
> ½ cup ice
>
> ½ cup unsweetened green tea
>
> Juice of ¼ lemon; add zest (scraped peel) to boost vitamin power
>
> 1 nickel-sized slice of peeled ginger
>
> 1 tsp honey

SOUP FOR LUNCH

WINTER SQUASH SOUP

> 1 9-oz package of frozen winter squash, such as butternut or acorn
>
> 2 cups hot water
>
> 1 bouillon cube (chicken or vegetable)
>
> Salt to taste

Place the ingredients in a blender, puree, then heat in the microwave.

Note: For variety, substitute pureed frozen spinach, peas, or asparagus for the squash. To increase the calorie count, substitute 1 cup of unsweetened almond milk or add ½ cup of soft tofu to the water.

In addition to the soup, you may have 1 cup of brown rice topped with half an avocado, 2 tsp slivered almonds, a drizzle of olive oil and a squeeze of lemon juice. Add soy sauce and sesame seeds if desired.

EVENING MEAL

1 cup brown rice

2 cups steamed chopped kale, chard, broccoli, cauliflower, or beet
   greens, seasoned with lemon juice, olive oil, or soy sauce

½ cup boiled lentils or cooked black beans, seasoned with garlic, salt,
   and pepper

If you want, you can also enjoy 1 cup of My Grandfather's Soup.

MY GRANDFATHER'S SOUP

1 quart water

1 yellow onion, sliced in half

½ bag baby carrots or carrot sticks

2 celery stalks

1 or 2 chicken bouillon cubes

2 boneless, skinless chicken breasts, cubed

2 nickle-sized slices ginger

2 to 3 oz each of the following:

> Goji berries or Chinese lycii berries (strengthen the liver and kid-
> neys)
>
> *Astragalus* root (bolsters your immune system)
>
> Codonopsis root (strengthens your vital energy or qi)
>
> Dioscorea root (Chinese yam root) (strengthens your lungs and
> kidneys)

Cover and simmer for two hours.

Note: Asian stores sell a prepackaged version of this soup with all these
Chinese spices packed together. It is known as Change of Seasons Soup and is
used to help people transition into the fall and winter without getting ill. At
my grandfather's house, we used it to boost our health when we felt we were
getting ill or worn down, and he regularly delivered it to neighbors and friends
who were not feeling well.

Masie's Mom's Incredible Tea

For a treat during this detox week or any other part of the diet, try this delicious tea!

Take an airtight tin of your favorite loose tea (rooibos tea or Ceylon tea work well) and add ½ cup of dried cherries to the tea leaves. The taste is stronger the longer the cherries are kept with the tea. When you brew the tea, make sure to get a few cherries in the cup. The cherries are delicious to eat after you've brewed your tea. Add a splash of milk and some almond or vanilla extract if desired. This is a great tea for before bed.

If you need a quick fix you can add a small amount of cherry preserves to a cup of tea for a sweet, fast treat.

Acknowledgments

As this is my first book and there are so many stories from my past that I have shared within it, the list of people to whom I am grateful is long. First and foremost, I would like to thank my patients for allowing me to be involved in their care. I enjoy sharing in their triumphs and helping them move to the next place in their personal wellness. They, in turn, reward me with new insights in how the mind and body intricately affect each other in often unanticipated ways.

Many people ask me how I became interested in integrative medicine. My interest was sparked by my maternal grandparents with whom I spent most weekends in the early years of my life. I am Chinese American and my grandfather, being the head of our family, was also the primary cook. My job was to assist him in the kitchen. His knowledge of herbs and medicinal soups was extensive and I learned much being his apprentice. I never would have been able to appreciate the value of traditional healers and their use of herbs had it not been for those early years with my grandparents. The support of my father, Curtis; sister, Sabrina; stepsister, Lindy; and half brother, Chris, has been tremendous and I thank them for being there in critical times when my energy was flagging, and for cheering me on while I wrote this book. I also would like to thank, though they have all passed, my stepsister Lori, mother and stepmother, Cynthia and Millie.

Living and working in another culture such as Micronesia, where traditional healers and elders in the community are valued and highly esteemed, planted the seeds for my questioning some of the things I learned in my Western medical training. The doctors and medical officers in the Public Health Service with whom I worked during my years in Micronesia—especially the practitioners who had been in service for many years away from the United States—were influential in shaping my understanding of how island life can be healing. In addition, I gained much insight in working with Dr. Victor Yano, a highly respected Palauan chief as well as a Western-trained medical physician. He modeled a Palauan form of an integrative medical practice at his private clinic long before the concept was formulated in the United States by fusing the wisdom of traditional indigenous Palauan practices and culture with conventional medicine. As we became friends, I observed firsthand how powerful the interaction between island family life and community can be in positively influencing health and well-being. I also want to thank all the Micronesian staff physicians, medical officers, and other healthcare professionals in Yap and Palau with whom I worked. Each made a point of giving so much of themselves and extending their friendship, making me feel like a welcome member of their community. In addition, many thanks to the Etpison, Kitalong, Yano, Soaladoab, and Beck families, who made me feel like family and have left their mark on this book.

If you really immerse yourself there, the Micronesian islands never leave your heart. That is why I joined my research partner, Dr. Michael Balick of the New York Botanical Garden, when he returned to Micronesia in 1998 to interview traditional healers and document how plants are used as medicine on Pohnpei and Palau. As of this writing, Dr. Balick and I (and the NYBG team) have now worked together on this project for more than a decade. I thank him greatly for his tireless effort in reviewing the countless essays, grant proposals, and articles that we have written together over the years. Though this is not an ethnobotanical book, our work together lent perspective to my understanding of just how much the pace of Western life and its values differ from others around the world.

Studying with Andrew Weil, and receiving formal training in integrative medicine at the Program in Integrative Medicine at the University of Arizona (PIM) set me on a trajectory that continues to this day. Over the years, Dr. Weil's support has gone far beyond the two years of my residential training in Tucson, Arizona. I am deeply moved by his generosity with his time and mentorship. I am also indebted to Victoria Maizes, Tieronna Low Dog, Randy Horowitz, Dean Emeritus James Dalen, Joseph Alpert, and other PIM faculty and staff for their support and generosity.

I would also like to thank those who contributed to my training at the PIM in those early years. Thanks to Tracy Gaudet, John Tarrant, Sue Fleishman, Colleen Growchowski, and the original "first gang of PIM four" classmates: Russell Greenfield, Karen Koffler, Wendy Kohatsu, and all the other residential "fellows." We had many visitors and faculty whose shared wisdom has found its way into this book. I would like to thank: Jon Kabat-Zinn, Saki Santorelli, Rachel Naomi Remen, Harriet Beinfield, Effrem Korngold, Linda Russek, Gary Schwartz, Iris Bell, Fredi Kronenberg, Mark Blumenthal, Paul Stamets, Tom Newmark, Paul Schulick, Mark Hyman, Dean Ornish, Vic Sierpina, Mary Jo Kreizer, Susan Folkman, Mary Hardy, Dave Rakel, and others whom, though not mentioned by name, equally shaped my enthusiasm for carrying on the integrative medicine torch.

The birth of the Continuum Center for Health and Healing (CCHH) in New York continues to be another huge gift of life experiences. I have been there since the center's inception and I would like to thank all the clinicians, support staff, and especially Woodson Merrell, Barbara Glickstein, Cathy Schaffer, and Ben Kligler—who have realized the dream of creating a more humanistic healthcare environment and have been supportive of my efforts to write this text. Also, a very special thanks of appreciation to Bill Sarnoff, for his generous mentorship and support in helping the center come to be at Beth Israel Medical Center. Working at the center is a community effort, and I count all the doctors, expert healing arts practitioners, nurses, and office staff among my blessings as well. My assistant, Troy Garriga, was instrumental in keeping me at the right place at the right time in chaotic moments while I was writing. A special shout-out to Bonnie Everhart for scheduling assistance and support.

Friends and colleagues in the healing arts were also very instrumental in keeping the project alive. I would like to thank Ruth Nerken for her help in developing conceptual clarity in preparing the book, and Kelly Campbell and Alison Bradley for photography support. Others who also helped clarify the vision are Susan Main, Shelley Berc, Alejandro Fogel, Annie Fox, Rusty Bergen, Selma Rondon, Andrea Balick, Karen Reivich, Andrew Shatté, Sonja Lyubomirsky, Todd Kashden, Jan Bruce, Beth Dill, Elishiva Gordis, Carol Ann Valentino, Toddi Gutner, Susan Stautberg, Eddie Weiner, Rita Foley, and all the Belizian Grove members. Thank you all for your support. Thank you to Dewey and Xena for your endless enthusiasm. And thanks to Adelle Lutz for sharing your soup secret—so simple and so delicious. I also want to thank Gideon Pine for assistance and Steven and Kimberly Rockefeller, Jr., for their friendship and support on the book and help in finding location shots at the Rockefeller State Park.

Two individuals broadened my perspective tremendously in thinking about stress and its greater impact; I wish to thank Rabbi Joseph Teluskin and Rabbi Simon Jacobson for their generosity in helping me in this regard.

Ina Yalof is a great writer who also became a great friend. Her talents are on display on every page of this book.

Every literary endeavor has behind it great editorial and writing support. This project was no exception. To my publishers and support help at Random House, Gina Centrello, Marnie Cochran, Tom Perry, Sanyu Dillon, Avideh

Bashirrad, Stacey Witcraft, Matthew Schwartz, Andrea Sheehan, Ken Wohlrob, Sally Marvin, and all—thank you. It was a pleasure having all of you guiding me along the way. Also special thanks to Paul Bogaards, Sheila O'Shea, and Will Murphy.

InkWell Management has been another beacon of support. Thank you to Michael Carlisle, Kim Witherspoon, Elisa Petrini, Rose Marie Morse, Alexis Hurley, Peter, Ethan, Nathaniel, Charlie, Julie, Rosemarie, Jennie, and Libby (who is now in law school) for your support, humor, and good cheer. Masie Cochran, thanks for sharing your mother's incredible cherry tea—that was such a great gift from both of you and I am grateful for your generosity.

The last thank-you is saved for my literary agent, Richard Pine, a tremendously insightful, humorous, and patient person whom I can also call a cherished friend. Thank you for the many candid and thoughtful conversations sprinkled with humor. I look forward to more books and conversations.

Notes

INTRODUCTION

1. Demetria Gallegos, "Americans Spend More Time with Computer Than Spouse." *The Denver Post* online, January 24, 2007. http://www.denverpost.com/search/ci_5075438

CHAPTER ONE

1. B. S. McEwen, "Protective and Damaging Effects of Stress Mediators," *New England Journal of Medicine* 338 (1998):171–79.
2. N. Adler et al., "Relationship of Subjective and Objective Social Status with Psychological and Physiological Functioning: Preliminary Data in Healthy White Women," *Health Psychology* 6 (2000):586–92.
3. N. Adler et al., "Socioeconomic Status and Health: The Challenge of the Gradient," *American Psychologist* 49 (1994):15–24.
4. Katherine Rosman, "BlackBerry Orphans," *Wall Street Journal,* page W1, December 8, 2006.
5. Research presented by Dr. Charles Nemeroff at the 161st Annual Meeting of the American Psychiatric Association. As reported in *NeuroPsychiatry Review* 9, no. 6 (2008).
6. B. Bower, "Well-Groomed Rodents Stay Cool, Calm: Individual Rat Response to Stress Influenced by Mother's Style of Nurturing," *Science News,* vol. 152, no. 11, p. 167, September 13, 1997.
7. R. M. Shansky et al., "Estrogen Mediates Sex Differences in Stress-Induced Prefrontal Cortex Dysfunction," *Molecular Psychiatry* 9, no. 5 (2004):531–38.
8. Dr. Avi Sadeh. Presented at the Association of Sleep Societies Meeting, June, 2001. As reported on the website Franklin Institute Resources for Science and Learning. http://www.fi.edu/learn/brain/sleep.html
9. A. Vgontzas et al., "Middle-Aged Men Show Higher Sensitivity of Sleep to the Arousing Effects of Corticotropin-Releasing Hormone Than Young Men: Clinical Implications," *Journal of Clinical Endocrinology & Metabolism* 86, no. 4 (2001):1489–95.

10. A. Vgontzas et al., "Chronic Insomnia Is Associated with Nyctohemeral Activation of the Hypothalamic-Pituitary-Adrenal Axis: Clinical Implications," *Journal of Clinical Endocrinology & Metabolism* 86, no. 8: 3787–94.

11. Stanley Coren, PhD. "Sleep Deprivation, Psychosis, and Mental Efficiency." *Psychiatric Times* Vol. 15 No. 3 (March, 1998) www .psychiatrictimes.com

12. K. Spiegel et al., "Impact of Sleep Debt on Metabolic and Endocrine Function," *Lancet* 354, no. 9188:1435–39.

13. Yamin Anwar, "Sleep Loss Likened to Psychiatric Disorders," as reported on UC Berkeley News website. http://berkeley.edu/news/media/ releases/2007/10/22_sleeploss.shtml

14. E. Epel et al., "Accelerated Telomere Shortening in Response to Life Stress," *Proceedings of the National Academy of Sciences* 101, no. 49:17312–15.

CHAPTER THREE

1. G. S. Kienle and H. Kiene, "The Powerful Placebo Effect: Fact or Fiction?" *Journal of Clinical Epidemiology.* 50, no. 12 (1997):1311–18.

2. The Kirtan Kriya Singing Exercise 2003 Research Study was a joint project between the Alzheimer's Research and Prevention Foundation and the Amen Clinic of Newport Beach, California, affiliated with the University of California at Irvine. For more information go to: http://www .alzheimersprevention.org/research.htm

3. T. Field et al., "Lavender Bath Oil Reduces Stress and Crying and Enhances Sleep in Very Young Infants," *Early Human Development* 84, no. 6:399–401.

4. Christopher R. K. MacLean et al: "Effects of the transcendental meditation program on adapative mechanisms: Changes in hormone levels and responses to stress after four months of practice." *Psychoneuroendocrinology* Volume 22, no. 4, (1997):277–95

5. Jin, P. "Efficacy of Tai Chi, brisk walking, meditation, and reading in reducing mental and emotional stress." *Journal of Psychosomatic Research,* 36, no. 4, (1992):361–69.

6. From the website of Pacific College of Oriental Medicine "A 2002 NIH survey found that about 8.2 million American adults have used acupuncture, and that 2.1 million had used it in the previous year." www.pacificcollege.edu/prospective/profession.html

7. T. Field et al., "Massage Therapy Reduces Anxiety and Enhances EEG Pattern of Alertness and Math Computations," *International Journal of Neuroscience* 86 (1996):197–205.

CHAPTER FOUR

1. The American Psychological Association's 2007 *Stress in America* survey.
2. Melissa Gotthardt, "The Miracle Diet," as reported in *AARP Magazine,* January/February 2008.
3. J. A. Vinson, J. Proch and P. Bose, "MegaNatural® Gold Grapeseed Extract: In Vitro Antioxidant and In Vitro Human Supplement Studies," *Journal of Medicinal Food* vol. 4, (2001):17–26.
4. This survey was commissioned by the Food and Mood Project. Information was found online at www.foodandmood.org. The information was moved over to Mind's website when the Food and Mood Project closed in January 2009. The new website is: http://www.mind.org.uk/foodandmood/
5. J.E. Alpert, and M. Fava, "Nutrition and Depression: The Role of Folate." *Nutrition Review* Vol. 55, no.5, (1997):145–9.

CHAPTER FIVE

1. H. Wahbeh et al., "Binaural Beat Technology in Humans: A Pilot Study to Assess Psychologic and Physiologic Effects," *Journal of Alternative and Complementary Medicine* 13, no. 1 (2007): 25–32.
2. W. Whang et al., "Physical Exertion, Exercise, and Sudden Cardiac Death in Women," *Journal of the American Medical Association* 295, (2006):1399–1403.
3. Tim Web, "Double Calories Burned with Five Minutes of Exercise!" on the website Medical Health Reports (2005).
   http://www.medhealthreports.com/General/Fitness/Double-Calories-Burned-With-Five-Minutes-Of-Exercise!.html

CHAPTER SIX

1. Lionel Tiger, *Optimism: The Biology of Hope* (Cary, N.C.: Kodansha America Inc., 1995).
2. Joshua Wolf Shenk, "What Makes Us Happy?" *The Atlantic,* June 2009.

3. D. D. Danner et al., "Positive Emotions in Early Life and Longevity: Findings from the Nun Study." *Journal of Personality and Social Psychology* 80, no. 5 (2001):804–13.

4. L. W. Poon et al., "Individual Similarities and Differences of the Oldest-Old in the Georgia Centenarian Study," *The Gerontologist* 29, no. 43 (1989).

5. Barbara Fredrickson, *Positivity* (New York: Crown, 2009).

6. Nicholas Wade, *The Science Times Book of Language and Linguistics* (Guilford, CT: Lyons Press, 2000), p. 175.

7. "University of Maryland School of Medicine Study Shows Laughter Helps Blood Vessels Function Better." The results of the study, conducted at the University of Maryland Medical Center, were presented at the Scientific Session of the American College of Cardiology on March 7, 2005, in Orlando, Florida. http://www.umm.edu/news/releases/laughter2.htm

8. Sonja Lyubomirsky, *The How of Happiness: A New Approach to Getting the Life You Want* (New York: Penguin, 2008).

9. Roger Emmons, *Thanks!: How the New Science of Gratitude Can Make You Happier* (Boston: Houghton Mifflin Harcourt, 2007).

10. Karen Reivich and Andrew Shatte, *The Resilience Factor: 7 Keys to Finding Your Inner Strength and Overcoming Life's Hurdles* (New York: Broadway, 2003).

CHAPTER SEVEN

1. L. Smith-Lovin and M. McPherson, "Social Isolation in America: Changes in Core Discussion Networks over Two Decades," *American Sociological Review* 71 no. 3 (June 2006):353–75.

2. Jim Rubens, *OverSuccess: Healing the American Obsession with Wealth, Fame, Power, and Perfection* (Austin, TX: Greenleaf Book Group, 2008).

3. Rob Haralson, "Hi There. I'm the Internet. I Like Romantic Dinners, Long Walks on the Beach and . . . ," *Research Policy's* online journal, 463 (October 2007). Poll released by 463 Communications and Zogby International. http://www.463.blogs.com/the_463/2007/10/hi-there-im-the.html

4. L. Hawkley et al. "Loneliness Is a Unique Predictor of Age-Related Differences in Systolic Blood Pressure," *Psychology and Aging,* vol. 21 (March 2006): 152–64.

5. S. Pressman et al., "Loneliness, Social Network Size, and Immune Response to Influenza Vaccination in College Freshmen," *Health Psychology* 24, no. 3 (2006):297–306.

6. Sheldon Cohen and Edward P. Lemay: "Why Would Social Networks Be Linked to Affect and Health Practices?" *Health Psychology* Vol. 26 No. 4:410–417 (2007).

7. Chris Crowley and Henry Lodge, "How Friendships Keep You Healthy," *The Daily Star*.net, January-February, 2007. http://www.thedailystar.net/magazine/2007/01/02/ls.htm

8. Howard Bloom, "Isolation, The Ultimate Poison," in *The Lucifer Principle: A Scientific Expedition into the Forces of History* (New York: Atlantic Monthly Press, 1997).

9. T. Jackson, "Social Support and Health Practices Within Community Samples of American Women and Men," *Journal of Psychology* 140, no. 3 (2006): 229–46.

10. A. R. Mitchinson et al., "Social Connectedness and Patient Recovery After Major Operations," *Journal of the American College of Surgeons* 206, no. 2 (2008): 292–300.

11. Gabrielle LeBlanc, "Five Things Happy Women Do," *O: The Oprah Magazine,* March 2008.

CHAPTER EIGHT

1. M. E. McCullough et al., "Religious Involvement and Mortality: A Meta-Analytic Review," *Health Psychology* Vol. 19, No. 3 (2000):211–22.

2. "Religious Involvement Linked to Good Health," National Institute for Health Research. As reported in the online journal Life Positive. http://www.lifepositive.com/mind/psychology/stress/mental-health.asp

3. N. Krause, "Gratitude Toward God, Stress, and Health in Late Life," *Research on Aging* 28, no. 2 (2006):163–83.

4. Rosalind Wiseman, *Queen Bees and Wannabes: Helping Your Daughter Survive Cliques, Gossip, Boyfriends, and Other Realities of Adolescence* (New York: Three Rivers Press, 2003).

5. Fyodor Dostoevsky, Constance Garnett (trans.), *The Brothers Karamazov* (New York: Modern Library, 1996).

6. Allan Luks, *The Healing Power of Doing Good: The Health and Spiritual Benefits of Helping Others* (New York: iUniverse.com, 2001).

7. Joan Borysenko, *Minding the Body, Mending the Mind* (Boston: Addison-Wesley, 1987), p. 176.

8. Dan Custer, *The Miracle of Mind Power* (Englewood Cliffs, N.J.: Prentice-Hall, 1960).

9. Alvaro Fernandez, "Meditation on the Brain: A Conversation with Andrew Newberg" on the website Sharp Brains: The Brain Fitness Authority, December 4, 2008. http://www.sharpbrains.com/blog/2008/12/04/meditation-on-the-brain-a-conversation-with-andrew-newberg/

10. Herbert Benson and Miriam Z. Klipper. *The Relaxation Response* (New York: Harper, 2000).

11. Harold G. Koenig, Michael E. McCullough, David B. Larson, *Handbook of Religion and Health: A Century of Research Reviewed* (New York: Oxford University Press, 2001).

FINAL THOUGHTS : LIVING SERENITY

1. Pine, Arthur, *One Door Closes, Another Door Opens: Turning Your Setbacks into Comebacks* (New York: Delacorte Press, 1993).

APPENDIX

1. Julia Child, *From Julia Child's Kitchen* (New York: Gramercy, 1999).

2. Mollie Katzen, *The Moosewood Cookbook* (Berkeley, CA: Ten Speed Press, 1992).

Index

About the Author

Roberta Lee, M.D., is Vice Chair of the Department of Integrative Medicine, Director of Continuing Medical Education, and Co-Director of the Fellowship in Integrative Medicine at Beth Israel's Continuum Center for Health and Healing (CCHH) at Beth Israel Medical Center in New York City.

She attended George Washington University Medical School and, following the completion of her residency in Internal Medicine, she served as a U.S. Public Health Service physician in Micronesia for five years. For the past ten years, she has travelled back to Micronesia as the ethno-medical specialist on an inter-disciplinary team of biologists, ethno-botanists, ecologists, and conservationists studying a cross-section of cultural and botanical influences on health, healing, and the promotion of wellness in chronic disease.

Dr. Lee is one of the four graduates in the first class from the Program in Integrative Medicine at the University of Arizona conducted by Andrew Weil, M.D. She lives in Chappaqua, NY.